Stigma and
Mental Illness

Stigma and Mental Illness

Edited by

Paul Jay Fink, M.D.
Medical Director, Philadelphia Psychiatric Center;
Chairman, Department of Psychiatry
Albert Einstein Medical Center
Philadelphia, Pennsylvania

Allan Tasman, M.D.
Professor and Chairman
Department of Psychiatry and Behavioral Sciences
University of Louisville School of Medicine
Louisville, Kentucky

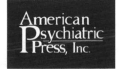

American
Psychiatric
Press, Inc.

Washington, DC
London, England

Copyright © 1992 American Psychiatric Press, Inc.
ALL RIGHTS RESERVED
Manufactured in the United States of America on acid-free paper.
94 93 92   4 3 2
First Edition

American Psychiatric Press, Inc.
1400 K Street, N.W., Washington, DC 20005

Library of Congress Cataloging-in-Publication Data
Stigma and mental illness / edited by Paul Jay Fink, Allan Tasman. —
   1st ed.
      p.   cm.
   Includes bibliographical references and index.
   ISBN 0-88048-405-5
   1. Mental illness—Public opinion—Congresses. 2. Psychiatry—Public opinion—Congresses. 3. Mental illness—United States—Public opinion—Congresses. 4. Psychiatry—United States—Public opinion—Congresses. 5. Stigma (Social psychology)—Congresses.
   I. Fink, Paul Jay. II. Tasman, Allan, 1947-   .
   [DNLM: 1. Attitude to Health. 2. Mental Disorders. 3. Patient Advocacy. 4. Psychology, Social.   WM 100 S8554]
   RC454.4.S75   1991
   306.4'61—dc20
   DNLM/DLC
   for Library of Congress   91-26135
                                                                                CIP

British Library Cataloguing in Publication Data

A CIP record is available from the British Library.

Contents

Contributors

William R. Breakey, M.D.
Associate Professor, Department of Psychiatry and Behavioral Sciences
Johns Hopkins University School of Medicine
Baltimore, Maryland

Louann Brizendine, M.D.
Clinical Faculty
Stanford University Medical School
Oakland, California

Francis T. Cullen, Ph.D.
Professor, Criminal Justice Program
University of Cincinnati
Cincinnati, Ohio

Norman Dain, Ph.D.
Professor of History
Rutgers, the State University
Newark, New Jersey

Howard Dichter, M.D.
Director, Outpatient Services
Philadelphia Psychiatric Center
Philadelphia, Pennsylvania

Leah J. Dickstein, M.D.
Associate Dean for Faculty and Student Advocacy
Professor of Psychiatry and Behavioral Sciences
University of Louisville School of Medicine
Louisville, Kentucky

William R. Dubin, M.D.
Deputy Medical Director
Philadelphia Psychiatric Center
Philadelphia, Pennsylvania

Norman S. Endler, Ph.D., F.R.S.C.
Professor of Psychology
York University
Toronto, Ontario, Canada

Amerigo Farina, Ph.D.
Department of Psychology
University of Connecticut
Storrs, Connecticut

Paul Jay Fink, M.D.
Medical Director
Philadelphia Psychiatric Center;
Chairman, Department of Psychiatry
Albert Einstein Medical Center
Philadelphia, Pennsylvania

Edward H. Fischer, Ph.D.
Connecticut Valley Hospital
Middletown, Connecticut

Pamela J. Fischer, Ph.D.
Department of Psychiatry and Behavioral Sciences
Johns Hopkins University School of Medicine
Baltimore, Maryland

Jeffrey D. Fisher, Ph.D.
Department of Psychology
University of Connecticut
Storrs, Connecticut

Glen O. Gabbard, M.D.
Director, C. F. Menninger Memorial Hospital;
Training and Supervising Analyst
Topeka Institute for Psychoanalysis
Topeka, Kansas

Krin Gabbard, Ph.D.
Associate Professor
Department of Comparative Literature
State University of New York at Stony Brook
Stony Brook, New York

Robert Gibson, M.D.
President and Chief Executive Officer
Sheppard & Enoch Pratt Hospital
Towson, Maryland

Mary Gullekson, Ph.D.
San Francisco, California

Donald P. Hay, M.D.
Associate Clinical Professor of Psychiatry
Department of Psychiatry, University of Wisconsin Medical School;
Executive Director, Association for Convulsive Therapy
Milwaukee, Wisconsin

Lisa D. Hinz, Ph.D.
Private Practice
Indianapolis, Indiana

Esso Leete
Denver, Colorado

Harriet P. Lefley, Ph.D.
Department of Psychiatry
University of Miami School of Medicine
Miami, Florida

Bruce G. Link, Ph.D.
Psychiatric Epidemiology Training Program
Columbia University
New York, New York

The Mad Hatters
Theatre for the Understanding of People
With Special Needs or Disabilities
Kalamazoo, Michigan

Jerold Mirotznik, Ph.D.
Associate Professor
Brooklyn College
Brooklyn, New York

Michael F. Myers, M.D., F.R.C.P.(C)
Clinical Professor
Department of Psychiatry
University Hospital, Shaughnessy Site;
Clinical Professor, Department of Psychiatry
University of British Columbia
Vancouver, British Columbia, Canada

Mark J. Mills, M.D., J.D.
Clinical Professor of Psychiatry
Department of Psychiatry;
Director, Program in Psychiatry and Law
University of California, Los Angeles (UCLA) School of Medicine
Los Angeles, California

George Mora, M.D.
Clinical Professor of Psychiatry
Albany Medical College
Poughkeepsie, New York

Gerald Nestadt, M.D.
Department of Psychiatry and Behavioral Sciences
Johns Hopkins University School of Medicine
Baltimore, Maryland

Glen Peterson, M.D.
President, East Bay Psychiatric Association
Oakland, California

Alan Romanoski, M.D.
Department of Psychiatry and Behavioral Sciences
Johns Hopkins University School of Medicine
Baltimore, Maryland

Bennett Simon, M.D.
Clinical Associate Professor of Psychiatry
Cambridge Hospital
Cambridge, Massachusetts

Herzl Spiro, M.D., Ph.D.
Professor of Psychiatry
University of Wisconsin Medical School
Milwaukee, Wisconsin

Elmer Struening, Ph.D.
Associate Professor of Public Health
Columbia University;
Chief, Epidemiology of Mental Disorders Research Unit
New York State Psychiatric Institute
New York, New York

Allan Tasman, M.D.
Professor and Chairman
Department of Psychiatry and Behavioral Sciences
University of Louisville School of Medicine
Louisville, Kentucky

Introduction

This book grew out of the 1989 American Psychiatric Association annual meeting, the theme of which was "overcoming stigma." The problem of the stigma against mentally ill persons and their caregivers has been a difficult and perplexing issue that has affected every aspect of the field of psychiatry. Patients' willingness or unwillingness to be treated, the inability to pay for treatment, and the unwillingness of people to have mentally ill persons living near them or working in their companies have combined to form the most powerful antitherapeutic forces that mentally ill individuals face.

For decades, psychiatrists have been subjected to jokes and ridicule because of their seemingly mysterious and incomprehensible ways of understanding the human mind and human passions. The complexity of mental illness and its often bizarre presentation are distressing to the layperson. One way an individual or society often deals with something that is frightening and distressing is to segregate it, alienate it, and set it outside the framework of one's personal society. This process results in stigma against patients and providers, and has manifold meanings and ways of expression.

We define stigmatization of mental illness as the marginalization and ostracism of individuals because they are mentally ill. This ostracism often also extends to the families of mentally ill individuals and to the professionals who treat persons with mental illness. Stigma associated with mental illness can cause those afflicted to delay seeking treatment or to conceal the illness in an attempt to escape the shame and isolation of being labeled "disturbed" and "other." Insurance benefits often do not adequately cover mental health care, and fear of losing health insurance coverage deters people from obtaining help. Employment and housing discrimination are just two other examples of the devastating effects that stigma can have on the lives of individuals. To combat the destructive effects of stigmatization, professionals must recognize and work to overcome the stigma associated with mental illness in our society.

This work is our attempt to draw together a sourcebook for mental health professionals on the problem of stigma by including a range of materials from scholarly studies to first-person accounts. Our goals are to sensitize mental health professionals to the pervasiveness of stigmatization of mentally ill persons and to inspire their understanding of the effects that this social and cultural problem has on patients, family members, and the caregivers themselves. Because professionals involved in treating mentally ill persons can either inadvertently perpetuate stigmatization or work to eliminate it through behaviors and attitudes, the first step in attempting to overcome stigma is to consider ways in which we can educate ourselves and the lay public concerning both the subtle and overt ways in which stigma works. The chapters in this book are intended to facilitate this awareness of the problem and to delineate possible approaches to solving it. Lay readers also will find much material in these pages to help them understand the roots and manifestations of a long-standing social and cultural problem. Ultimately the destigmatization of mental illness will be accomplished when people understand what psychiatric disorders are and believe that they are treatable.

The 1989 annual meeting included a large number of presentations dealing with this subject; the theme of overcoming stigma was a major track throughout the scientific sessions. Many papers presented were of high quality, and it was gratifying to find so many professionals struggling with this issue in one form or another.

This book grew out of our immediate awareness that this topic had a community of scholars and a constituency of millions who are interested in not only overcoming stigma but also having a greater understanding of how it develops, what it means, and why it is so persistently pervasive. The collection of chapters for this book involved some difficult choices, particularly because there were so many excellent papers presented at the 1989 sessions. The book is not intended to be a comprehensive presentation of all aspects of the subject of stigma and mental illness, but rather an introduction to a problem that is the subject of ongoing research.

The book begins with an overview of the effects of stigma on psychiatric treatment. The remainder of the volume is divided into four sections.

The first section contains personal accounts that convey powerful information about the effects of stigma on the individual and family. The introductory brief presentation by Dr. Gullekson, the letter from a resident whose name has been withheld, and the chapter by Esso Leete, a former mental patient, all express the passions involved when one experiences stigma either firsthand or through the experience of a family member.

In Section II the authors address the historical view of stigma against mentally ill persons. Chapters are included on ancient Greece and the medieval and Renaissance periods. In other chapters the authors address specifically the Devon Asylum, as an illustration of how attitudes toward treatment of mental illness can change, and the perspective of American Christianity. These chapters were selected to provide background for our modern concerns about stigma and how our perceptions of mental health and mental illness have or have not changed through the centuries. Much important research on the historical aspects of stigma is ongoing, but we were unable to include all that we wanted to include. Our intent was to give some perspective on the problem of stigma, but to focus primarily on the here and now.

Societal issues are the focus of Section III, and in these chapters the authors address stereotypes from several different angles: the stigma perceived by patients, the effects of stigma on homeless mentally ill persons, and cinematic stereotypes that contribute to the stigmatization of psychiatrists. The stigmatized family of the mentally ill person is discussed in another chapter, and helping the doctor's family to fight stigma is the subject of the final chapter in this section.

In Section IV the authors address several institutional issues, including the stigma of mental illness for medical students and residents, problems faced by deinstitutionalized psychiatric patients, the psychiatric hospital and the reduction of stigma, the stigma of electroconvulsive therapy, and the stigmatization of psychiatrists who work with chronically mentally ill individuals.

The concluding chapter is a contribution from the Mad Hatters that provides a different perspective on the issues discussed in other chapters.

This book serves as a collective call to action by over 30 authors who are determined to see a turnaround in the way in which human beings dehumanize one another. We are pleased with this book not only because it represents the success of the American Psychiatric Association annual meeting in 1989 and the extraordinary interest and excitement over the issue of destigmatization, but also because it is a continuation of our interest and research into the causes and underlying problems of stigma.

Paul Jay Fink, M.D.
Allan Tasman, M.D.

Chapter 1

Effects of Stigma on Psychiatric Treatment

William R. Dubin, M.D.
Paul Jay Fink, M.D.

S tigma against mentally ill persons is so pervasive that it affects every aspect of their lives. It brings with it a multitude of problems, from insurance, to housing, to jobs; stigma stops patients from getting the best treatment, or at times from getting any treatment at all.

Historically, people with psychiatric illnesses have been stigmatized. Such stigma pervades writings from medieval to modern times. Mental illness was once thought to be related to being possessed with demons. In more recent times, while such concepts are no longer prevalent, patients with mental illness continue to be viewed as constitutionally weak, dangerous, and responsible for their own plight. It is interesting to take special note that although patients with other illnesses such as tuberculosis or epilepsy were once stigmatized, patients with these illnesses no longer suffer the social ostracism that they once experienced. However, prejudice against patients with mental illness persists unabated.

Stigma Related to Professional Attitudes

There are a multitude of factors that explain why stigma against mentally ill persons has been so persistent. People find it difficult to accept behavior that is so different from the norm. Often patients with psychiatric illness manifest bizarre behavior that is just too frightening to accept or acknowledge. Psychiatrists and mental health workers often perpetuate the biases of laypersons. For example, nonpsychiatric physicians downplay the concept of mental illness being a biological illness. This bias is frequently conveyed in the physician's statement to his or her patients: "You're not crazy. You don't need to see a psychiatrist. I'll send you to a psychologist or social worker."

In hospital settings, psychiatrists and mental health workers perpetuate the concepts of stigma. Psychiatric units are established with the expectation of bizarre, aberrant, and out-of-control behavior. For instance, when patients come into a psychiatric hospital, the system is structured for them to earn privileges. Programs are not designed with the focus of making the hospital experience as normal as each person's everyday routine outside the hospital. Instead, patients are placed on various levels of restriction until they demonstrate that they are not dangerous.

Normalcy has to be proven before patients are given the same rights that they would possess outside of the hospital. For example, in the hospital many patients have to be in bed by 9 or 10 o'clock. Yet most people do not go to bed at this time. Those patients who do not comply are given sleeping medications or seen as noncompliant and resistant to treatment.

Another routine is that of mealtimes. In most hospitals, patients eat three meals in 8 or 9 hours. They have breakfast at 7:30 A.M., lunch at 12:00 P.M., and dinner at 4:30 or 5:00 P.M. In life, most people do not eat meals that close together; yet if patients say, "I don't want to eat supper tonight," or, "I don't want to go to breakfast this morning," we tend to categorize them as being uncooperative or as possessing an unrealistic sense of entitlement.

Other examples abound. Following admission to a medical hospital, patients are allowed a telephone and television in their rooms. In a psychiatric facility, this is not done. Obviously, at certain levels of illness when patients are suicidal, this is not feasible; yet when patients are past these stages, they still cannot have a telephone or television in their rooms. The inherent assumption on the part of the caregivers is that a psychiatric patient with an in-room telephone will misuse the phone, that is, make threats, harass family members, or use the telephone cord to inflict self-injury (i.e., make a suicide attempt).

A corollary example of how we stigmatize patients is in the organization of a psychiatrist's office. In many offices, patients are permitted to come in one door and then leave through another door for fear someone will see them. While this may respect their privacy, there is no precedent in any other area of medicine in which patients leave through the back door after seeing their physician. Again, we acknowledge, pander to, and rationalize this stigma.

Often psychiatrists are put on the horns of a dilemma, having to weigh the realities of stigma in society versus the therapeutic efforts to instill a sense of normalcy in our patients. For example, a 21-year-old patient asks: "Doctor, I want to go to medical school. Should I put on my application that I have seen you in psychotherapy for two years?" What is the response? It is a difficult decision.

Stigma of Other Physicians

Many physicians developed jaundiced views of psychiatry because in medical school their psychiatry rotation was in a state hospital or in a Veterans Administration hospital. As a result of this experience, they developed the belief that all psychiatric illness is chronic and that psychiatry has very little to offer patients. In their own practice, they do not equate their middle- and upper-middle-class patients with the patients they encountered in these hospital settings and proceed under the notion that their patients could not possibly suffer from the same illness or disease as the patients whom they took care of when they were medical students.

A phenomenon all psychiatrists have experienced is that of receiving consults in a hospital and having to explain to irate patients why they are there because the attending physician never told them they were going to consult a psychiatrist.

Stigma Related to Treatment

We often tend to stigmatize many of our treatments. Electroconvulsive therapy is an effective, at times lifesaving treatment modality that until recently has been repeatedly stigmatized by the lay press and by members of the psychiatric profession. As a result, many patients do not avail themselves of this extremely effective treatment and develop chronic depressions that do not respond to medication but would respond to electroconvulsive therapy if they would allow themselves to receive this treatment. Even the use of psychiatric medications causes concern. For example, a colleague of one of the authors was taking antidepressant medication and did not want anyone to know. In a discussion, he stated that were he in psychotherapy he would not be ashamed of psychotherapy and would probably take great pride in it. However, he felt that taking a medication for depression would not be acceptable among professional colleagues because it suggested some type of inherent weakness or inability to function without chemicals. In fact, he shared the bias that if he were only "strong enough" he would be able to overcome his depression without the use of medication.

Social Stigma

Perhaps the most pernicious of all myths is that of the dangerousness of psychiatric patients. While less than 3% of mentally ill patients could be categorized as dangerous, 77% of mentally ill people depicted on prime-time television are presented as dangerous. This perpetuates the mythology that if one is mentally ill, one is by definition dangerous. This myth is further perpetuated by the sensationalistic headline news both in newspapers and on television when murders are committed by former mental patients. Interestingly, no reporter is interested in the failures of the mental health treatment system that has often allowed these patients to go for long periods of time untreated and, in many instances, be forced out of hospital settings into the community against the recommendations of psychiatrists.

To the average citizen, these stereotypes of bizarre, potentially dangerous psychiatric patients are further ingrained as one walks along any major urban street and views the devastating effect of psychosis on many homeless individuals. The fact that society lets these people remain untreated further trivializes the importance of treatment and ignores the significant advances that have occurred in psychiatric diagnosis and treatment over the past 25 years. In contrast to these patients, if someone is bleeding or passed out on the street, would everyone continue to walk by? Yet under the rubric of civil rights we are willing to let someone who is suffering from severe mental illness lie on the street often to the point of freezing to death. The fact that we leave these people on the street makes an implicit statement that we really do not care about mentally ill persons and that society is not willing to accept this group of people.

A major problem in combating stigma is the lack of public awareness of the advancements that have occurred in psychiatry over the past 25 years. Too often perceptions are still those of hospitals being "snake pits" or that all patients are going to be treated with five-day-a-week psychoanalysis. The lay public has little appreciation of how effectively psychiatrists can treat affective disorders, anxiety disorders, or control the symptoms of schizophrenia. There is vast ignorance in the public sector as to the advances that have been made in psychiatry, which in combination with the pervasive stigma would prevent people from seeking and obtaining help. Additionally, the myth that there is something about the American character that says we should have strength to be able to take care of ourselves continues to take precedence over the concept that mental illness is a biological illness which is treatable and not self-induced.

Family and Stigma

Families have continually borne the prejudicial effects of stigma. While it is true that the patients suffer because of the painful symptoms of mental illness, the stigma of this illness becomes like an infectious disease to members of the family. Often the family unrealistically feels blamed and responsible for having brought on the illness. This burden is further perpetuated by certain members of the psychiatric community who continue to suggest that biological illnesses are really a result of dysfunctional, inadequate parenting. The development of various groups like the National Alliance for the Mentally Ill is overcoming this outdated misinformation by providing a national forum to educate the public as to the etiologies of mental illness. In the past, families were accustomed to being passive and accepting whatever psychiatrists told them. To the benefit of psychiatry and to the credit of the family, they no longer have assumed this docile role and are willing to ask pointed questions and demand reasonable answers.

Mental illness can destroy families. Couples may get divorced if they have a family member who is mentally ill. Often family funds are seriously compromised in the effort to take care of a mentally ill member. Because the lingering myth of the family being at fault continues, many families focus exclusively on mental illness being a brain disease, leaving out the mind. Psychiatrists must play an important role with these families, emphasizing that treatment involves not only biological intervention but also social rehabilitation and environmental manipulation.

Psychiatrists inadvertently abet stigma by refusing to meet with the family based on the issue of confidentiality. It is important that psychiatrists develop greater flexibility and understand the needs of families and try to work a compromise so that while acting in the patient's best interest, they can also be an important source of nurturing and support for the family.

Stigma and Insurance

Inadequate insurance coverage for mental illness is a well-known issue. The majority of insurance companies have severe limitations. For inpatient treatment of a psychiatric illness, reimbursement rarely exceeds $50,000 lifetime coverage. In contrast, open heart surgery or renal dialysis patients have almost unlimited coverage. Outpatient coverage for psychiatric illness is even more restrictive, often with high copayments, up to a limited amount, and once that amount is reached, reimbursement ceases. This discrimination has gone on for many years and continues even with the advent of health maintenance organizations (HMOs), which appear to be more egalitarian in their approach. Yet, restrictive clauses prevent patients with chronic mental illness from enrolling in many HMOs.

Mental illness in this country historically has been paid for by state government. This has been due in part to the fact that communities would not do it because of the problems of stigma and opted to leave mentally ill persons adrift. The public system involves a whole series of complex funding issues. Rules and regulations, often unrealistic, provide a maze of impediments to treatment. Funding sources are varied, each with its own regulations. This situation ultimately results in care being provided in a haphazard, piecemeal fashion. The steady erosion of state funding throughout the country has worsened an already untenable situation.

Insurers believe that psychiatric illnesses are chronic, untreatable illnesses that are going to undermine the financial well-being of their companies. Similarly, they have a bias against psychiatrists and feel that every psychiatrist is untrustworthy and that they are going to treat the patient until the last day of insurance coverage. However, they never comment about the overutilization of electrocardiograms, chest X rays, and the other unnecessary tests that physicians may use to obtain results on their patients. The psychiatrist, the patient, and the mental illness are all indiscriminately lumped together.

Stigma and Advocates

The number of advocates for the mentally ill is exponentially increasing around the country. The National Alliance for the Mentally Ill, the National Depressive and Manic Depressive Association, and the National Mental Health Association are examples of grass-roots organizations that are bringing together people to fight aggressively for more funding, better services, and more adequate treatment facilities. This perhaps has been one of the most significant developments in the past 100 years regarding a movement toward destigmatization. The effects of public education in reducing stigma can also be seen in the number of people who come for outpatient treatment. The number of firms that utilize Employee Assistance Programs is increasing. Educational programs that are being developed by the American Mental Health Fund are beginning to increase public awareness of the myths of mental illness. The American Mental Health Fund has sent out over a quarter of a million booklets in response to inquiries about an advertisement that it ran. The American Psychiatric Association has had a major role in destigmatization by producing 100,000 calendars with the 10 warning signs of mental illness and distributing them all over the country. Additionally, radio and TV spots of the 10 warning signs have significantly increased caller inquiries to the psychiatric societies, indicating that there are people responding to educational information. The Depression, Awareness, Research and Treatment (DART) initiative that is being sponsored by the National Institute of Mental Health is another major public education program. This program takes on special importance because it is an effort on the part of the federal government to educate the entire country about depression. As breakthroughs in psychiatric research occur, these will also help to consolidate the gains in reducing stigma and increase the public's awareness and appreciation of the possibilities of psychiatric treatment.

Perhaps one of the most extraordinary public education efforts was the "Moods and Music Concert." A manic-depressive professional worked with major orchestras in this country to organize a concert featuring the music of five manic-depressive composers. Listening to the music of geniuses like Handel, Schumann, Berlioz, Debussy, and others, we realize that sometimes people whom we stigmatize as inferior are superior. It is a real eye-opener to become confronted with one's own prejudice. How could anybody call Handel a mentally ill person? When one listens to the *Messiah*, a person does not identify the composer as mentally ill. Handel happened to have a mental illness. How would people feel if they began to realize that some of the most important people in the arts and sciences have had definable, diagnosable mental illnesses?

One of the bright spots involving the issue of stigma has to do with research. Traditionally, federal investment in research for mental illness has been low; however, it does appear that after several years of decline the support of psychiatric research is increasing. This is an optimistic sign.

Conclusion

The obligation of all psychiatrists is to try to reorganize treatments and treatment programs so that we do not end up being stigmatizers ourselves. Could we treat our patients when they are in the hospital as if they still have all of their rights? We must acknowledge our own prejudices against mentally ill persons whether they are outpatients or inpatients. This is the most difficult issue for any professional to confront. How can we reduce the amount of stigma perpetrated and perpetuated by us as professionals? Psychiatrists must be aware of the advances that have been made in specificity of treatment, must practice at the highest standards of care, and must constantly improve the standards by which they practice. If we can help patients recover or significantly improve their functioning, we have helped reduce the stigma. We can all alert our colleagues to the obligations they have in paying attention to the problem of stigma, paying attention to their own prejudices against mental illness, paying attention to many of the issues that they never think about when they see one patient at a time. Stigma is a pervasive national and international problem, an insidious problem that is destructive to families, mentally ill patients, and the profession of psychiatry. We can and we must change this course.

The Experience of Stigma

Chapter 2

Stigma: Families Suffer Too

Mary Gullekson, Ph.D.

The contribution of Dr. Mary Gullekson, a psychologist from California, is among the most articulate statements of the nature and quality of stigma against mentally ill persons that we have ever read. Hers is a brief but very powerful contribution. Dr. Gullekson's experiences are not unusual, but her ability to put them into a brief statement expresses the depth of feeling that families have with regard to their mentally ill children, parents, and siblings.

My brother was 12 years old when he was diagnosed as paranoid schizophrenic and committed to the state hospital. I was eight. Needless to say, our lives changed forever.

To speak about siblings of mentally ill persons is to speak of ambivalence, ambivalence that exists at the deepest levels—that of a sibling relationship stretched to the limits of connection. It is to speak about loss and grief. It is about bonding with affection and bonding without affection. It is about polarization, love and hate, affection and fear. It is about wanting to be close and a survival need to be distant.

For the most part, intensity is the prime adjective of description. The pain burns. A sibling once known is now lost. This pain is intensified even more by the confusion and overwhelming feelings of the parents. Anger pervades, anger at the situation and anger at the perceived helplessness of the self and of the parents. A sibling is an integral part of what happens between the parents and the ill child. Mental illness affects the whole family. It is a catastrophic event for which a developing child has few skills to cope with.

Certainly not the skills to deal with stigma.

For me stigma means fear, resulting in lack of confidence. Stigma is loss, resulting in unresolved mourning issues. Stigma is not having access to resources, resulting in lack of useful coping skills. Stigma is being invisible or being reviled, resulting in conflicts regarding being seen. Stigma is low-

11

ered family esteem and intense shame, resulting in decreased self-worth. Stigma is secrecy, resulting in lack of understanding. Stigma is judgment, resulting in lack of spontaneity. Stigma is divisive, resulting in distrust of others. Stigma is anger, resulting in distance. Most importantly, stigma is hopelessness, resulting in helplessness. This all adds up to decreased potential, of self and for others.

David is now 50 years old. I know little of who he was. Memory does not permit. I know him only as he is: a man of courage, intelligence, maturity. Perhaps not in the usual sense, but then his life has not been usual, has it? He has fought for the right to live outside the walls, and he has fought the good fight.

It is comforting to me today to see so many people who care about stigma and will devote time and energy to it. Thank you. It helps.

Chapter 3

A Letter From a Resident

The following letter was sent to one of the editors (P.J.F.) because of his long-standing interest in the problem of stigma against mentally ill persons. The horror of these experiences is neither unusual nor unexpected. Nevertheless, it is testimony to the prejudice all of us have against mentally ill individuals, including all of those trained as caregivers, family members, siblings, and even the mentally ill persons themselves. This letter is another articulate statement of stigma as it is felt by a real person—as it is experienced by someone who has a mental illness. As long as we continue to treat mentally ill persons as if they will never be as good as we are, as if they can be helped but not cured, as if they are lesser human beings who by virtue of their illness must be placed at a lower level and thereby dehumanized, we will perpetuate stigma. Changing our own prejudice may be the most critical and important thing that we have to do during the next decade in order to entirely destigmatize persons with mental illness.

December 15, 1988

Dear Dr. Fink:

I am a PGY-IV resident in psychiatry. I am also mentally ill. I am bipolar and a recovering alcoholic. It has been difficult and trying at times. Sometimes I feel as though it is too much and I should reevaluate my goals. I did not know of my mental illness when I began my pursuit of medicine. Your emphasis on overcoming stigma has done as much for my heart and soul as years of therapy and medication. I would like to tell you about my residency experience and how you have influenced me.

I have been hospitalized twice during my residency, both [times] during my second year. The episode of illness was precipitated by a 2,000-mile move away from my friends and family. I became depressed while doing an inpatient rotation at a private hospital. My work suffered, but not nearly as

---

Published by permission. The author requests anonymity.

13

much as I did. Upon returning to work, every mistake I made seemed like a death sentence. All my movements were checked, friendly conversations at the nurses' station no longer included me, and invitations for after-work get-togethers quit coming. The looks and comments under the breath were almost too much for me to bear. I became toxic on my medication and had to return to the hospital. I felt angry and betrayed, not only by those around me, but by my medication. I used vacation time for hospitalization in order to keep up with my fellow residents. I was asked to leave the residency program. For some naive reason I was expecting words of support, offers of help, or maybe some needed time off. I refused to take an offer for a possible position in research. I realized then that I was on my own and whatever happened I had to do it alone. I also wondered if I was wrong. Maybe I couldn't do it. Maybe I was harmful to my patients, my profession, or myself.

I have survived the deaths of my parents in the past 18 months. After each death I was watched closely for signs of deterioration. Displays of normal grieving were something I could not risk. After the second death I was advised by my attorney to make a last will and testament. Xeroxing copies of the will at work was interpreted by fellow residents as a suicidal gesture, and I was reported to the administration. I was devastated. When I suggest ideas at residency meetings they are ignored. When I privately tell my chief resident the same idea and she introduces it, it is usually accepted. My self-esteem suffers, but I tell myself that good ideas are enough, recognition shouldn't matter. Sometimes I even believe that lie. I do not think anyone in my residency is personally against me. I believe they have made and continue to make the best decisions available to them. I doubt they are aware of how I perceive their actions. They truly do not know. God bless them.

My brother is my only family left. Like most lay people he says I can pull myself together when I want to. He tries to be supportive but he will not leave me alone with his three-year-old son. When developing new friendships I say nothing of my disease to avoid the stigma I've learned soon follows. I also feel the burden of discrimination against psychiatrists. I want to be good for my profession by being a good physician and a good person. I think others will view me as "crazy like all psychiatrists" if they know that I have been ill. This thinking has been fostered by the treatment I have received from fellow psychiatrists. I continue in treatment to deal with these issues, but it is not just my problem.

During the last three years I have won an original paper competition sponsored by the state psychiatric association. I have one article in press and another in review. My PRITE [Psychiatry Resident in Training Examination] scores are consistently one and sometimes two standard deviations above the average. With the assistance and recommendations of the psychiatric residency where I completed my first year, I have been accepted into a fellowship in consultation-liaison psychiatry.

I draw my strength from old friendships. I receive hope and perspective from my patients as I help them in their struggle towards health. My inspiration comes from rare individuals who not only understand my perspective but know what to do next. You are one of these people. After listening to you speak on the enigma of stigma and reading many of your publications, I'm learning how to effectively fight back against stigma. The shame of my illness is disappearing and I am developing pride in my life.

Thank you for your leadership. If there is ever any way I can repay you please do not hesitate to ask.

Chapter 4

The Stigmatized Patient

Esso Leete

In this chapter, Esso Leete, who has struggled with schizophrenia for over 20 years, shares her personal feelings and observations about the meaning of stigma.

More than by any other one thing, my life has been changed by schizophrenia. For over 20 years I have lived with it and in spite of it, struggling to come to terms with my illness without giving in to it. Although I have fought a daily battle, it is only now that I have some sense of confidence that I will survive my ordeal.

Let me give you some background on myself, my history, if you will. I am the eldest of three children. My father was in the Army and we moved every few years, including to Germany. I was shy and slow to make friends, and these frequent uprootings were extremely difficult for me; I sorely missed the predictable routines, stable friendships, consistent schools, and familiar houses that others enjoyed.

We returned to the United States for my senior year of high school, which is when I became ill. I didn't know it at the time (and I think others denied it), but looking back I can see the changes. Except for participation in sports, I had always been more comfortable by myself, and in my senior year I became increasingly withdrawn and sullen. I felt alienated, lonely, and angry for no apparent reason. Everyone was so distant from me; there seemed to be a huge gap between me and the rest of the world, including my family. I watched dispassionately as my two younger sisters matured, dated, shopped, and shaped their lives, while I seemed stuck in a totally different dimension.

I graduated with honors from high school. It was expected that I would get a scholarship, and I did. When I reluctantly went off to college, however, I was without my family for the first time and totally unprepared for life away from home. Although I was able to perform my school work, I remained isolative; I had no close friends, and as time went on I spoke to virtually no one. I found myself drawing pictures of Van Gogh and writing poetry in classes instead of taking notes. I saw myself in a foreign world that I could not always translate. At one point I believed I was on Venus. I forgot to eat and began sleeping in my clothes. Even routine things like taking a shower rarely occurred to me.

Toward the end of that first semester I had my initial acute psychotic episode. At the time I did not understand what was happening, and it was extremely frightening. One night walking alone on a beach my perceptions suddenly shifted. The intensifying wind became an omen of something terrible, trees and bushes bent threateningly toward me, and tumbleweeds chased me. I was running but making no progress. When I finally reached my dormitory after what seemed like hours, I was exhausted, confused, and hearing voices for the first time. Later that week I had other similar experiences, still not comprehending that I was out of touch with reality as others know it. That reality had given way to the multiple realities with which I would now live.

One day soon thereafter I returned from classes and was surprised to find my father in my dormitory room, my bags packed and waiting at the door. Someone must have notified him of my condition, for he had come to take me away. He had been advised that I was ill and should be treated in a hospital; this was my first psychiatric admission. Diagnosis: Schizophrenia. Prognosis: Extremely guarded. I was treated with medications and released after a few months. I have since been hospitalized 15 times, the longest hospitalization lasting a year. I have had twice as many doctors. I have had 10 diagnoses (most of them variants of schizophrenia), been prescribed nearly 20 medications, and had almost every kind of therapy imaginable, including four-point restraint and seclusion "therapy," as well as insulin coma therapy concomitant with electroconvulsive therapy (ECT). In other words, I have been treated with everything for everything.

Although physical abuse and neglect of mental patients is no longer rampant, we continue to be faced with a less visible but no less brutalizing psychic cruelty: stigma. It has been my experience that there is nothing more devastating, discrediting, and disabling to an individual recovering from mental illness than stigma, which *Webster's* (in an older edition) defines as "the scar or brand left by a hot iron on the face of an evildoer." This brand is a mark of disgrace, of shame. It signifies that an individual is different, someone to be avoided. Such a tainted person is seen as unbelievable and therefore untrustworthy. And persons who cannot be trusted must be feared.

Throughout history, no group has been as maligned as people with psychiatric disorders, beginning with negative expectations regarding our character and our conduct. We have suffered long from widespread ignorance and the effects of a prejudice that is pervasive. I have personally learned about this the hard way. You understand stigma firsthand when:

* You are given insulin coma therapy and ECT without being consulted or informed because your psychiatrist and your family assume you are too ill to understand.
* Your college refuses to readmit you after discharge from the hospital because you now have a history of mental illness.
* You are denied a driver's license because you are naive enough to answer their questionnaire truthfully.
* A general hospital emergency room doctor brusquely explains, after reading in your chart the diagnosis of "residual schizophrenia," that your fever, nausea, and vomiting are "all in your head."
* Your friends decide they need to develop other relationships on learning of your past troubles and treatment.

Stigma is an ugly word, with ugly consequences. Yet not everyone is judged equally; studies show that there are certain personal characteristics that influence the extent of our social rejection. Males are more heavily stigmatized than females. The lower the social class, the more likely a mentally ill person is to be excluded from the community. The public rejects disturbed behavior that is socially visible, especially if it is violent. In our culture it is far less socially acceptable to be troublesome, disruptive, or bizarre than it is to be detached or withdrawn. A history of hospitalization is more stigmatizing than a history of outpatient care.

There are countless examples of stigma, a serious problem for everyone afflicted with a mental illness. One of the most significant, in my opinion, is that the mentally ill cannot find meaningful work. Job applications still weed us out by asking if we have ever been hospitalized, if we are taking any medication, if we have a chronic illness. When we have spent time in a hospital, we must find creative ways of accounting for our time. When we are taking medications and experiencing noticeable side effects, we must have a plausible explanation for these.

Even if we are successful in obtaining employment, we are often still discriminated against. A friend of mine had finally secured a job and worked for about 3 months. At the end of that time he felt he had become friends with his employer, so he mentioned to him one day that he was diagnosed as manic-depressive, assuring him that he was now on medication and doing very well. The employer responded that although he would not fire him, he would in the future pay him only $5.00 per hour instead of the $8.00 per hour originally set. Can you imagine how this individual felt, the message that this conveys?

The prejudices held with regard to mentally ill persons as employees are profound, which is why it is estimated that at any given time only 10% to 30% of those with a psychiatric history are employed. Yet work is one of the most beneficial therapies that we have. Just having a job, along with its corresponding structure, imparts the following benefits to me: It gives me something to look forward to every day, a skill to learn and to improve. It is my motivation for getting up each morning. My hours are passed therapeutically as well as productively. There is a built-in way to socialize with others, but in a place where this is not the main expectation or criterion, thereby making it less threatening. As I successfully work, I become increasingly self-confident and independent; my self-image and self-esteem are bolstered. I feel I am self-supporting like others, and I have money to buy what I need as well as extras. (This is never true on SSI.) I feel important and grown up, which replaces my usual feelings of vulnerability, weakness, and incompetence. Indeed, I believe that meaningful employment is essential to the recovery process.

Another problem for us is locating housing. Typically, when my halfway house in Denver attempted to build a new facility, neighbors came from far and wide to protest and humiliate us and were successful in opposing our application. In addition, our history of mental illness prevents us from fair hearings in divorce and child custody hearings. Security clearance is virtually impossible. In short, we are literally branded for life.

Socially, we are ostracized. Most of us live quite lonely and isolated lives. People continually avoid us and do not want to be with us—and we know this. Making and keeping friends, always a difficult task for us, becomes harder still when others discover our background. With each social encounter we must consciously decide whether or not to tell about ourselves, whether or not to lie, always fearing the embarrassing discovery of our pasts if we cannot pass as "normal." When I do not want to speak to someone next to me on an airplane, I have discovered that all I need to do is in some way mention my disability (even that I am traveling to make a speech about it) and this individual becomes absolutely mute for the remainder of the trip.

We hear jokes about psychiatrically labeled individuals like ourselves on a daily basis. Personally, I cannot laugh at such insensitivity; often I feel like crying. Living with a chronic mental illness is no laughing matter. Increasingly, this kind of poor taste is also found on many commercial products, another indication of the public's ignorance of the serious impact of a mental illness on one's life.

Insurance companies continue to discriminate against mentally ill persons with biased reimbursement schedules. When I tried to get insurance coverage through my group plan with the state, Blue Cross/Blue Shield informed me that my schizophrenia was a preexisting condition and that I would not be covered for the first year if I had been receiving psychiatric treatment. To overcome this I tried not seeing my psychiatrist for the requisite 6 months prior to coverage, perhaps not the best solution. And, as you know, there is continuing indifference from those involved with public policy and research funding for mental illness.

One of the most painful events that has happened to me occurred some months ago. The Colorado Civil Rights Act prohibits discrimination on the basis of race, creed, color, sex, age, national origin, ancestry, and physical handicap, but provides absolutely no protection for mentally ill persons. Therefore, discrimination against individuals with mental illness has been legal under Colorado law.

Recently a bill was introduced that would add "mental impairment" to the definition of "handicap," thereby extending the existing prohibitions against discrimination in housing, employment, public accommodation, and discriminatory advertising to include those persons who are mentally disabled, including those with a mental illness. We have tried every year to achieve this addition in the law, but unsuccessfully! I am outraged by this. It really hurts to be told, in legislation, that we are second-class citizens, not worthy of these rights. Fortunately, these rights have now been signed into law, although there are no monies for enforcement until the year 1991. I am not proud of Colorado citizens that it has already taken 10 years.

In addition, the mental health system has failed us; there is nobody more prejudiced against persons with mental illness than the psychiatric profession. Mental health professionals themselves often perpetuate negative attitudes toward mental illness, both blatantly and in more subtle ways. This probably sounds harsh, so let me explain. In general, psychiatry, the system with responsibility for the reintegration of patients, is stigmatizing in terms of its reluctance or inability to acknowledge our capabilities, which has a multitude of serious repercussions for those of us under its care.

Let me give some examples of behaviors I have encountered from the psychiatric profession. Not too long ago I attended an open house at a local mental health center and was having a pleasant conversation with a psychiatrist until I mentioned that I was a consumer. Quickly he muttered, "I've got to go now," turned his back, and walked away. I was in midsentence.

Even the psychiatric hospitals do not always offer the kind of assistance and humane care we need. Staff attitudes are reflective of their own ignorance and prejudices. When it was my word against someone else's, a someone with no history of mental illness, I had no credibility. At one point I had been, probably incorrectly, rediagnosed with a borderline personality disorder, and staff related to me only with reference to this. It did not matter that I had had a diagnosis of schizophrenia consistently for 20 years; it did not matter that I was plagued by fear and auditory hallucinations; it did not matter that what I probably needed was a medication consultation—none of these things mattered because the staff was too busy responding to me based simply on my new diagnosis. To their minds I was acting out, not being terrorized by voices; to their minds I needed seclusion and restraint, not medication. Maybe I am too close to the anger and pain I feel around this to be objective, but it certainly seems like an aspect of the worst kind of stigma when a patient is devalued to the point that ongoing reports of psychotic symptoms are viewed as mere manipulation, and then treated as such.

Just recently I experienced another traumatic bout of hospitalization. I was taken to the emergency room of Denver General Hospital by ambulance because I had become withdrawn and mute after being threatened and intimidated by police officers. When we arrived inside, staff asked me to follow them down the hall, which I compliantly did. I was feeling better and had already decided not to do anything that would result in my being detained or admitted. However, as I was quietly sitting on the gurney per their instructions waiting for them to communicate with me, the two ambulance attendants and two hospital staff members suddenly grabbed and shackled me by chains to the gurney. I had not been threatening, assaultive, loud, or demanding. In fact, I had to this point said nothing. I was not even evaluated to see whether or not I needed this form of "protection." My feeling is that they made their decision to place me in four-point restraints based on the fact that I was a mental patient and thus dangerous. To me this is another example of just how widespread the stereotypes are of mentally ill persons, even extending to presumably trained professionals.

One of the most common examples of deeply rooted and entrenched negative perceptions about mentally ill individuals held by professionals is in the vocational arena. Because it seems inconceivable to mental health professionals that we are capable of holding employment, we are relegated instead to something called "day care treatment." Day care is for the children of working parents, not for adults, not for us. It is demeaning and says much about how psychiatrists view our relationship with them and our potential. And what do we do in "day care"? Often nothing but sit around, drink coffee, and endlessly smoke cigarettes. We can do this in our own apartments, and often do rather than attending the center. No wonder.

I type medical records for a state hospital in Denver as my occupation, and I have had the opportunity many times to see these attitudes that reflect the perceived inadequacies of persons with mental illness. For example, I was told by one psychiatrist who neglected to note Axis IV and Axis V on his report that "it doesn't matter anyway because all of our patients are chronic patients and they aren't going to get better." It is quite common for psychosocial histories to state flatly that "vocational assessment is not warranted now or in the future." How do mental health professionals know that? Are psychiatrists prophets? No. Psychiatrists do not know what will happen in the future, to what extent we will recover, or our capabilities. Instead of working with us to build on our assets and to help us learn coping mechanisms, professionals many times see us as beyond repair and hopeless, not worth expending much time and energy on in terms of treatment.

Do you realize how devastating this negative perception of our prognosis can be to us in our struggle to recover? A poor prognosis colors every aspect of our lives. And if we have been able to establish an alliance and working relationship with you our doctors, we take what you think seriously. We trust you, we believe you. If you think that mental patients cannot function, cannot work, cannot recover, we sense this and often our hope is shattered and we will not even attempt recovery. Your set of expectations of us as low-functioning is thus self-reinforcing and self-perpetuating, and becomes a self-fulfilling prophecy.

Many of the behaviors of professionals actually promote stigma for patients. There is a lack of client choice in our treatment plans, our medication management, and our disposition after discharge. There is an insistence by the system that we do not know what is best for us and therefore need guardians and parents to make choices for us, even when we are not legally certified as incompetent. Clearly, mental health systems do not perceive that one of their duties should be the empowerment of the client, not enslavement. In addition, confidentiality, originally begun as a means of protecting people from stigma, actually ends up promoting it. Medical and psychiatric illnesses are seen as different classes of illnesses and receive different treatment. There is much more shame experienced when one is diagnosed with a mental illness than with a physical disease, and the toll we suffer in terms of self-esteem, self-image, and self-confidence is far worse. We must strive to increase the community's acceptance of those with mental illness. As one class of the poor and disenfranchised in this country, we ask that others recognize our needs and differences and respect them. If we receive the care we deserve, we can return to being productive members of our communities, and this will assist us in our ongoing efforts to overcome stigma.

Of course, we must first stop expecting someone else to "fix" us. This task falls to each of us alone, for no one else can really make us better. We must approach this task very seriously, conscientiously working to battle stigma and to put our lives back together. Not until I was ready to take responsibility for myself, including management of my illness, did my recovery really begin. As I began to defeat the inner stigma I experienced, I felt strong enough to attack the mistaken views of the public regarding the mentally ill and to put them in perspective. All of us must separate the disease from its victims.

I am proud to have been asked to prepare this chapter. All too often I have found professional presenters at psychiatric meetings speaking about the views of mentally ill persons on certain issues. Even in this way we are discounted, for we who are most involved and know best our own feelings and opinions are not consulted or asked to present on panels with professionals. If we are allowed to speak at meetings we are isolated out into one particular day, "Patient Day," instead of being integrated into the whole program, and attendance is woefully low. And, of course, continuing medical education credit is less for attending these workshops than for other workshops, once again concretely demonstrating how much worth mental health professionals attribute to our experience. We are left out of the mainstream, our abilities and expertise ignored, by the very people who should be trained to recognize our unique talents and the contributions we could make to the field. Isn't it about time that both the plight and the potential of individuals with mental illness are recognized?

What would the role of the mental health system be if it had a genuine interest in seeing us reintegrated into our communities as functional and contributing members? Why is there such resistance from the system to take on a strong rehabilitative flavor? Why does the mental health system so desperately want to keep us on its rolls? Is it the money? Is it because of fear of abandonment and rejection? I don't know, but my feeling is that we have a right to this recovery. How many have heard me speak and have trouble reconciling the fact that I am labeled a "CMI" and doing what I am doing and conclude that I must be misdiagnosed? If you believe that individuals with a chronic mental illness can never get well, and if I am able to make this speech, then that is obviously sophistry. Please do not expect the worst from us. Please reexamine those ingrained beliefs that we cannot recover, and please have hope for us.

Being treated with compassion and respect, as an individual with strengths and weaknesses instead of a mental patient who can never improve, is important. Hope is crucial to recovery, for our despair disables us far more than our disease ever could. The negative stereotype of our prognosis for recovery held by many professionals today and embodied in pejorative terms like "CMI" is very demoralizing and destructive to those of us struggling with a mental illness. We deserve better than to be labeled a treatment failure and dismissed. If we are "chronic," it is partly because mental health professionals have failed in their attempts to treat us, which is the inevitable outcome of having such a set of negative expectations.

I would like to conclude by mentioning one other disastrous effect of stigma. Because of stigma many of us are unwilling to admit our difficulties, understand and accept our illnesses, and actively learn how to cope with our symptoms. And we must overcome this stigma if we are to defeat our disorders. Positive feelings about ourselves can then be redeveloped, and we will once again view ourselves as the unique and worthwhile individuals we are. We will reclaim our personal validity, our dignity as individuals, and our autonomy.

In order to meet the challenge of our illnesses, we must change the image of who we are and who we can become. The paradox remains that only by learning to accept our limitations can we begin to discover our own unique possibilities. Although it takes time, we can overcome our illness and the myths surrounding it. We can compensate for our disabilities. We did not choose to be ill, but we can choose to deal with illness and learn to live with it. But we must—and will—shatter this stigma that now shackles us.

Historical Aspects of Stigma

Chapter 5

Shame, Stigma, and Mental Illness in Ancient Greece

Bennett Simon, M.D.

In this chapter the author provides a historical basis for the shame and stigma attached to mental illness. The attitudes and method of treatment described focus on Greece from the 5th century B.C. until the 2nd century A.D.; however, these views have persisted and can be seen in Western culture even today.

Dr. Simon investigates the history of the term "stigma" and shows how the concept became associated with mental illness in ancient Greece. He traces the centrality of shame, pollution, and erratic unpredictability in the stigmatization of mentally ill persons and demonstrates the way in which scientific and magical or religious practices attempted to reduce the stigma attendant upon illness. Awareness of the complex relationship between mental illness and other elements of Greek society has relevance to contemporary efforts to understand and eradicate stigma.

C onsiderable stigma was attached to mental illness in ancient Greece, and that stigma was intimately linked to the sense of shame. By focusing on the role of shame, we can best understand three aspects of mental illness in ancient Greece: 1) the culturally held attitudes and feelings toward mentally ill persons; 2) the theories of causation, especially medical and divine; and 3) the balance within the culture between extrusion of mentally ill individuals and the ritual means of cleansing and reinclusion. Medical theories of mental illness were attempts to reduce the stigma by asserting the supremacy of physiology over mythology. Black bile had less stigma than black motives. Fortunately, the Greeks were not so constrained by their theories that they failed to develop a pragmatic and flexible potpourri of methods for dealing with mental illness. The attitudes and methods of treatment described in this chapter, including the centrality of shame, focus on Greece from the 5th century B.C. until the 2nd century A.D. However, these attitudes have persisted in Mediterranean cultures to this day and can be seen to some degree in all of Western culture.

Stigma and Shame

In a historical examination of "stigma," it is important to consider the history of the term. It is a Greek noun (*stigma*), coming from roots that mean to make a point or a mark. It was probably most widely used to designate tattooing, whether decorative, religious, or to indicate ownership (such as on a slave). In earlier Greek usage, while this term could be used for a brand mark on a slave, it did not seem to have the automatic negative connotation it has acquired today. It had some usage in referring to wounds inflicted in military service, more like a badge of honor. In the New Testament and in early Christian Greek, the term stigma only gradually became associated with the wounds of Christ, which are not called stigmata in the Gospels. An important usage in late antiquity is that of a tattoo mark signifying that the person is dedicated to a particular god (i.e., a mark of service). When Paul writes, "I bear on my body the stigmata of Christ" (Gal. 6:17), he seems to refer to two metaphorical usages, the first being the sign of service to a god, and the second, the sense of a wound inflicted in the course of serving as a soldier of Christ. The more negative connotation of the term appears in Latin, where the Greek word is taken over, and metaphorically denotes a mark of shame or degradation, a mark placed on criminals or slaves so that they could be identified if they ran away. According to the *Oxford English Dictionary*, its clearly pejorative metaphorical use appears in the English in the late 16th and early 17th centuries.

Although the term stigma was not used in ancient Greece in relation to mental illness, there was considerable stigma attached to mental illness in Greek culture, and that stigma was intimately linked to the sense of shame. Despite a certain philosophical "romancing" with the concept of madness, and even religious awe sometimes attached to mental illness (e.g., epilepsy being known as "the sacred disease"), mental illness, especially if chronic, was regarded at best as undesirable and at worst as requiring that afflicted persons be shunned, locked up, or, probably on rare occasions, put to death. As in much of the world, both historically and today, where family and extended family units had a large share of responsibility for members in distress of whatever sort, most of those patients were cared for within the province, or the confines, of the family. There were no institutions for persons who were chronically (physically or mentally) ill.

Running like a red thread in all of the Greek sources on madness and mental illness are the themes of shame, loss of face, and humiliation. Concomitantly, the theme of *agon*, a battle, a competition, as marking much of human existence is ever present, and shame and its related distressing effects are especially prominent in relation to one's losing in one or another agonistic arena. The notion of pollution, that the madman is polluted and also can pollute (we shall see later how he might also heal), is interwoven with the sense of shame (Dodds 1951; Ducey and Simon 1975; Simon 1978). These were important aspects of ancient Greek culture and continue to be so in modern circum-Mediterranean cultures (Blum and Blum 1970; Lawson 1909/1964), and are in fact still part of all modern cultures. Let us turn then to several texts, more or less contemporaneous, from the latter part of the 5th century B.C.

Among the more morally neutral of ancient texts are the medical writings, in which we find observations about the role of shame in certain illnesses. In relation to epilepsy, the Hippocratic writer of "On the Sacred Disease" tells us something about the role of shame in the way patients regard the early warning, or premonitions, of an attack:

> Such as are habituated to their disease have a presentiment when an attack is imminent, and run away from men, home, if their house be near, if not, the most deserted spot, where the fewest people will see the fall, and immediately hide their heads. This is the result of shame (*hup' aischunes*) at their malady, and not, as the many hold, of fear of the divine. Young children at first fall anywhere, because they are unfamiliar with the disease; but when they have suffered several attacks, on having the presentiment they run to their mothers or to somebody they know very well, through fear and terror at what they are suffering, since they do not yet know what shame is. (Hippocrates 1922, xv, p. 171)

In this work, the author is arguing that the disease is no more or no less sacred than any other, and adduces either physiological or understandable emotional causes for the different aspects of the disease (Simon 1978; Temkin 1971). Here, the shame attendant upon having an attack explains a piece of the behavior (i.e., run and hide).

A good part of the opening chapters of "On the Sacred Disease" is devoted to belittling and ridiculing various magicians and charlatans who purport to know how to diagnose and treat the illness in terms of which deity has afflicted the poor epileptic person. The author is indignant at how such charlatans take advantage of suffering people, exploiting their clients' terror and ignorance for their own aggrandizement and profit. The list of superstitious and magico-religious and ritual pollution that requires purification is long. We get a good look in this treatise at the physician at work, simultaneously tooting his own horn—his is a real craft, and the others' are fake—and laying out theories of causality that clearly help to minimize the enormous burden of shame and loss of face attendant upon this affliction. Poseidon, Ares, Apollo Nomius, the Mother of the Gods—some of the deities allegedly causing one or another species of seizure—are not the true causes. Rather impacted phlegm in weak veins, overheated *pneuma* going to the brain, winds from particular directions, hereditary dispositions—these are the morally neutral causative agents that have replaced divine agents, who imply a larger measure of shame and/or blame.

In Greek tragedy, where there are the most memorable and "dramatic" presentations of madness, we find that the role of shame is quite prominent (Simon 1978; Starobinski 1974). In Sophocles' *Ajax*, the hero, Ajax, is deeply ashamed and enraged that he has lost out to Odysseus in the contest for the armor of the slain Achilles. The two chiefs of the Achaeans have made the award. To further the cause of Odysseus, her favorite hero, Athena drives Ajax mad, deluding him into thinking that a flock of cattle and sheep are an assembly of the chiefs of the Achaeans, so that he whips and slaughters animals he imagines are the two brothers, Agamemnon and Menelaus, and Odysseus himself, his hated rival. After Ajax has recovered from his madness and become aware of all that had happened to him, despite the urging of wife, son, and friends, he ends up, secretly, committing suicide. He is deeply ashamed and humiliated, afraid of further mockery and disgrace by the Greeks, unable to face his father, who obviously could not countenance a son who is in disgrace and stripped naked of all the rights and privileges of a heroic warrior. His wife's plea that it is shameful to leave an unprotected widow and an orphaned son also is of no avail. Explicitly, in terms of the text, shame is a major motive for suicide; implicitly (i.e., requiring some psychological interpretation of the character of Ajax) shame has already played a role in making him go mad. But here the Greeks are kind: it is not explicit that Ajax himself is responsible for his madness, but rather a somewhat capricious, or at least highly prejudiced, divinity, Athena, drove him mad. In terms of the play, the characters who love him can plausibly try to persuade him to forgive himself, because the shameful slaughter of the animals was not his own doing, as it were, but divinely prompted. The tragedy devolves around the fact that for Ajax this is not enough and still not acceptable. But we do get a glimpse of the extent to which the playwright expects that the audience will understand that an explanation of divine causation should be able to mitigate the overwhelming sense of shame and failure.

The value of explaining madness as a capriciously inflicted disease is again demonstrated in Euripides' *The Madness of Heracles* (Simon 1978). There we get a picture of a hero who is, for all intents and purposes, blameless and has been driven mad totally by some divine caprice. His madness consists of a delusional reenactment of some of his famous labors (from which he has just returned to rescue his wife and children in the nick of time), and he mistakes his children for the children of his worst enemy, Eurystheus. Heracles slays his wife and children and, when his madness remits, is intent on killing himself. The last portion of the play is devoted to a series of interchanges among Heracles, his father Amphitryon, and his friend Theseus, who is ultimately successful in dissuading Heracles from suicide. In the terms and language of the play, it is clear that the element of shame, as well as the loss of face, is a major part of Heracles' wish to kill himself (although certainly not the only motive), but the enduring friendship with Theseus is what enables him to survive the losses and the disgrace. Incidentally, his murderous fit is only stopped by Pallas Athena appearing and throwing a large stone that hits him in the chest and knocks him out. I believe that this is also an allusion to the practice of the stoning of madmen, to drive them away out of fear of their violence or fear of pollution, or perhaps even to act as a method of ritually healing them. In later antiquity a "stone for Heracles," known as the "saintly stone," was exhibited somewhere in the Peloponnesus and shown to tourists.

These vignettes already begin to show us a mixture of attitudes and a certain ambivalence in the culture toward mental illness. First, the Greek doctors who wrote about epilepsy did not concern themselves with whether it was a physical or psychical disease; distinctions between physical and mental illness were not sharply drawn, whereas the distinction between acute and chronic disease was quite important (Drabkin 1950). Indeed, it seems likely that the vast majority of cases of madness were of an acute sort and represented delirium in the course of a serious illness. The Hippocratic physicians in their clinical descriptions lump together accounts of delirium, pain, swelling, sparse urine, or copious and loose bowels, and so forth.

True, Plato begins to speak of "diseases of the mind" parallel to "diseases of the body," but he did this primarily to define a category of disturbances in living that would be amenable to correction and change by means of his philosophical methods (Lain-Entralgo 1970; Simon 1978). True, there is a rich metaphorical vocabulary of going crazy, but this is not to say this vocabulary implied a theory of purely "mental" causes as opposed to physical causes. Terms in current everyday English use, such as "a bad case of nerves" or "he's a real hothead," come closer to capturing popular Greek ideas about etiology. The humoral theory indeed grows out of popular and folkloristic ideas about body and behavior, and represents a systematization and formalization of these concepts. "He's in a bad humor" represents a living example of the use of a quasi-physiological explanation to explain, justify, or perhaps suggest treatment for a particular (transient) disturbed state. "Black bile," the cause of melancholy and some other dire diseases, is an extension of popular fantasies and beliefs about "blackness," combining black, or dark, substances emanating from the body and black moods, black thoughts, and black deeds. But "black bile" removes a certain measure of stigma from the person—it is more detached, more impersonal, more neutral. The tragedian's handling of the myth of Ajax's suicide can be usefully contrasted with a 4th-century physiologically based treatise on melancholy, the pseudo-Aristotelian work, *Problemata*, which begins with the query,

"Why are so many exceptional men melancholic?" (Klibansky et al. 1964; Simon 1978). This work describes mood swings due to the effects of hot or cold black bile, cases of which may end in suicide by hanging. Although mentioning a mix of historical and mythological figures, it totally glosses over issues of shame and loss of face. In the Greek worldview, a certain measure of shame, or disgrace, was attached to disease in general, and even to the most common of chronic diseases, growing old. Indeed, Greek medicine played a role in "naturalizing" and thereby making somewhat less shameful the whole state of being ill. In general, in Greek culture an affliction allegedly sent by the gods might be, alternately, a source of shame and humiliation, but the "fact" that it was caused by a god, and not by oneself, also served to mitigate the pain and the shame. Medical explanations created an even more favorable "balance of trade" in shame and disgrace by providing a more impersonal external causality.

Incidentally, the Greek doctors were part and parcel of the same cultural ambience of competition, shame, and disgrace at losing. It is difficult to say if Greek medicine was more of a "shame culture" than is modern medicine, for medicine has probably always been an intensely agonistic and "face"-oriented enterprise (i.e., importance placed on saving face). As such, these ancient doctors were very concerned about both their reputation and their own inner self-esteem. A fair amount has been written about how Greek doctors were careful to avoid taking on incurable cases, because it made their statistics, and their reputations, look worse. But the Hippocratic doctors were also "naturalizing" chronic and incurable illnesses as part of life, and not regarding them only as a source of shame for the doctor who cannot cure them. The doctor must be humble with the realization of the limits of his powers, but accordingly suffers less loss of face and reputation when he cannot cure.

In general, the methods and means of treatment available to Greek culture tried to deal with the elements of shame and pollution that seemed to accompany many, if not all, illnesses. If the culture labeled a certain condition as a divine possession, or possibly punishment, it had to provide as well the means to repair, atone, or exorcise. As such, medical theories and medical treatments for mental illness were only one means of regulating and controlling the distressing effects that perhaps played a role in the genesis of the disease, and certainly played a role in response to the disease. Thus, these same heroes who went mad, Ajax and Heracles, plus others such as Oedipus, had temples or small monuments erected at their purported burial sites, and these burial sites of mythic (and sometimes historical) warrior-heroes became healing shrines (see Knox 1964; Rohde 1925/1950). These mythic and mythohistorical figures, in some sense victims of the crushing weight of shame in Greek culture, could also become the source of healing and restitution. Overall, whether ritual, philosophical-dialogic, or medical means of treatment were employed, an important part was to "normalize" or destigmatize the patient.

One consequence of such a need is that in many cultures one sees the elaboration of a number of different theories and means of healing. Rather than seeing a multiplicity of theories as a feature only of highly developed or merged cultures, we might profitably view such a multiplicity as a propensity of many cultures to deal with the social press to provide an acceptable and shame-reducing framework to "socialize" an illness (Kleinman 1980). Greek culture certainly had such a multiplicity, and in the next section I wish to adduce two hypothetical cases to show the variety of means and rationales available.

The Pragmatic Potpourri of Treatments

Hypothetical Case 1

In late 5th-century B.C. Athens, a somewhat older man, in his early fifties, a father and grandfather, begins to become withdrawn, seclusive, and suspicious, and is drinking more than usual. He complains of sticking pains in his ribs on his right side and of his bowels not being right, and close family members think he is visually imagining things that are not there. He stops seeing his old "buddies," and one of them remembers that in the last conversation they had, he hinted at some difficulties of potency, and he reported being rebuffed in a recent attempt at a homosexual tryst with a teenage boy. However, these issues are only discussed, or gossiped about, among a small circle of friends. As the man gets more disturbed, people are more and more protective of him and do not wish to mar his reputation and increase his sense of shame by alluding to these difficulties.

This man might first go on a short trip outside of the city limits of Athens to a shrine of a hero, oddly enough called "Physician-Hero." There he might join with a small group of other worshippers and seekers of help, and offer some libation of honey and wine, poured upon the ground or into a vase, standing at the "grave-site" and uttering some appeal for help in his distress.

This visit to the shrine might be a prelude to his visiting a physician in a city the size of Athens. There would likely be local, resident physicians, although from time to time a prominent physician from another locale might pass through and be consulted. The physician would likely be interested in a detailed discussion of the man's symptoms and of his regimen of life: his place of residence, his travels, seasons of the year when his symptoms get better or worse, and a good deal of attention to his diet and exercise. There would be an inspection of the urine and of any phlegm or vomitus the patient might produce. The physician would quite likely make a diagnosis of a serious disease—a melancholic state. The pain under the ribs and near the liver would be called (literally) hypochondriachal ("under the ribs") and would be part of the symptom picture of melancholia, as would the withdrawal, suspiciousness, and possible visual hallucinations (Jackson 1985). There would be some discussion of the use of wine, especially the degree of dilution and the place of origin of the wine. There might well be some discussion of his dreams, and the dream material would be used to suggest occult disease somewhere in the body (e.g., dreams of the top floor of a building would suggest a problem in the head).

Treatment would consist of dosing, once or several times, with white or black hellebore, inducing either vomiting or bowel movements, or both. There might well be various fluids with which to wash, concocted of herbs and juices that would all be considered *cholegogues*, substances that help expel black bile. Foods low in black bile would be prescribed as well as some graded exercise regimen. It is quite possible that the physician would spend a fair bit of time explaining things to the patient, both the rationale for and the details of the treatment. The prognosis would be fair, especially if the doctor's orders are followed.

Concomitantly, or serially, the man might be considered by the family and neighbors as being possessed by some divine agency, especially if his behavior involved some fitful and erratic activity. He might be encouraged to participate in a ceremonial group, the *Korybantes*, a group of women and men (although the men tend to be more socially marginal, older, or deviant in other respects) who meet regularly for a kind of healing dance and trance ceremony. Depending on the degree of relief and/or pleasure obtained from the rhythmical dancing and ecstatic states, he might attend only once or twice, or he might become a regular member and indeed help to spread the good news about the group, and good rhythms, to others.

As word of the man's distress spread through the neighborhood, a variety of itinerant vendors of advice, magic rituals, special charms, and oracles predicting personal and collective future events, would find their way to his house. There would undoubtedly be some heated discussion among the family and neighbors about which of these is "authentic" and which a charlatan; nevertheless, there would be a steady stream of such people and their wares.

Again, depending in part on the degree of persistence and intractability of his symptoms, he might be brought by his family to a temple of Asclepius, perhaps one on the nearby island of Aegina. (The more famous one at Epidauros was in "enemy territory" in the Peloponnesus.) There, he would approach with a large group of other seekers of help and their families, and be exposed to a good deal of conversation and exchange of information about the healing successes, indeed miracles, of the god and his priestly interpreters. He might stop to read (or have read to him) some dedicatory inscriptions put up and donated by grateful patients who were successfully healed, detailing their illness and their healing experience through dream (Edelstein and Edelstein 1945). He would then undergo some ritual purification, receive instructions from the priest, have some contact with the snakes who are part of the sanctuary, and be escorted to a special area where he would sleep and receive a divinely inspired dream. The next morning he would relate the dream to a priest and have its full implications, including any particular instructions for prayer, medicine, and regimen, carefully explained. He and his family would have brought with them either an animal for donation—small or large depending in part on the family's wealth—or else a donation of silver or coinage.

If all else failed, and the man became much worse, and especially if he became violent, he would be secluded at home, and either family or people hired by the family would have to carefully watch over him and protect him from self-destructive tendencies as well as protect others from him. If he were not so violent, he might become a neighborhood curiosity, occasionally jeered at by boys in the street, and feeling a bit uncomfortable as passersby might spit, apotropaically, to ward off any evil to themselves from his look or from looking at him. At times, he might end up being pelted and stoned if he got too close for comfort to some of his fellow citizens.

In part, depending on the resources of the family, there might be numerous other attempts to find healing places or resources in other parts of Greece, or to eagerly seek one or another medical, magical, or divine practitioner who would be passing through Athens. It was entirely possible, then, as now, that the patient would not improve, and might go on to a lingering death by somehow becoming marasmic, wasting away, or that the patient might successfully commit suicide, perhaps by hanging himself.

One can see here how each of the steps in an attempt at healing is also an attempt to "normalize" or contextualize the man's illness, to make it part of some larger schema, and, in general, to remove or minimize any sense for him and for the family of personal responsibility for the illness. The family is motivated to support and try out all available modes of treatment, not only out of concern for the suffering of their relative, but also to reduce the shame and stigma inevitable in having a diseased and disordered family member.

Hypothetical Case 2

In later antiquity, say in 2nd-century A.D. Alexandria, or in Pergamon in Asia Minor, a similar picture appeared in an older man of modest wealth. The same modalities would be available, but there would be a much greater array of all of them. There would be a variety of physicianly opinions available, with numerous competing schools and practitioners. Were the patient well placed enough or wealthy enough to consult with Galen (a "philosophical physician") or one of his close associates, he might encounter some mixture of a physical exam (which would include more elaborate study of his pulse than in the preceding centuries, and a more sophisticated examination of sensory and motor nerve functioning) and a medically oriented history (Riese 1963). The timing and duration of previous melancholic episodes, as well as any intermittent states of elation or mania, would be scrutinized. In the course of discussion of various moral aspects of the patient's life, including relationships with his slaves, his wife, and his children, Galen would carefully note that certain topics seem to lead to an increased agitation in the patient, as evidenced, for example, by a change in the quality and rate of the pulse.

Galen would likely be quite emphatic in the superiority of his treatments to those of others, and would casually, but carefully, put down other physicians the patient had consulted, and any discussions he had had with philosophers of a somewhat different persuasion than that of Galen (who could be quite critical of the Stoics, for example). It is doubtful if the available methods of medicinal treatment would be substantially different from what had been available to our hypothetical patient in the 5th century B.C., but there would be a much more elaborate theoretical rationale for all of the treatments.

There would also be an array of magical and religious practices (Luck 1985). The available cults included those that worshiped Isis, Asclepius, Serapis, and Christ, as well as those using Jewish healing rituals or perhaps some early Gnostic rituals and treatments. The possibility of becoming a devotee of one or of more such cults was quite substantial, and the patient could well spend a good part of his remaining years in quest of peace and healing in the service of a god. Rituals involving one or another form of exorcism, driving out the alleged possessing *daemon* by prayers and curses, would be more widely available than in the 5th century B.C. (Dodds 1965). In all of these "modalities" of treatment, one could see an important element of incorporation or reincorporation into a community of an afflicted person who, by virtue of his or her illness, had become somewhat of an outcast.

Conclusion

The ancient Greek world was puzzled by the origins and treatment of severe mental illness, as we are today. The interwoven elements of shame, of pollution, and of the erratic unpredictability of the behavior of the severely mentally ill person contributed to stigmatizing that person and the illness. But, at the same time, the culture provided an array of practices, some considered "scientific" and some considered "religious" or "magical," but all designed to reduce the stigma attendant upon the illness. In the period we have described, from the 5th century B.C. to the 2nd century A.D., there was an expansion of means and modalities of treatment, but no fundamental change in either the efficacy or the motives behind the array of treatments.

References

Blum R, Blum E: The Dangerous Hour: The Lore and Culture of Crisis and Mystery in Rural Greece. London, Chatto & Windus, 1970

Dodds ER: The Greeks and the Irrational. Berkeley, CA, University of California Press, 1951

Dodds ER: Pagan and Christian in an Age of Anxiety: Some Aspects of Religious Experience From Marcus Aurelius to Constantine. Cambridge, UK, Cambridge University Press, 1965

Drabkin IE (ed): Caelius Aurelianus: On Acute Diseases and On Chronic Diseases. Translated by Drabkin IE. Chicago, IL, University of Chicago Press, 1950

Ducey CP, Simon B: Ancient Greece and Rome, in World History of Psychiatry. Edited by Howells JG. New York, Brunner/Mazel, 1975, pp 1–38

Edelstein EJ, Edelstein L: Aesclepius: A Collection and Interpretation of the Testimonies, 2 vols. Baltimore, MD, Johns Hopkins University Press, 1945

Hippocrates: Hippocrates, Vol 2. Translated by Jones WHS (Loeb Classical Library). Cambridge, MA, Harvard University Press, 1922

Jackson S: Melancholia and Depression: From Hippocratic Times to Modern Times. New Haven, CT, Yale University Press, 1985

Kleinman A: Patients and Healers in the Context of Culture. Berkeley, CA, University of California Press, 1980

Klibansky R, Panofsky E, Saxl F: Saturn and Melancholy. New York, Basic Books, 1964

Knox B: The Heroic Temper. Berkeley, CA, University of California Press, 1964

Lain-Entralgo P: The Therapy of the Word in Classical Antiquity. Translated by Rather LJ, Sharp JM. New Haven, CT, Yale University Press, 1970

Lawson JC: Modern Greek Folklore and Ancient Greek Religion: A Study in Survivals (1909). Introduction by Oikonomides ARN. New Hyde Park, NY, University Books, 1964

Luck G: Arcana Mundi: Magic and the Occult in the Greek and Roman Worlds. Baltimore, MD, Johns Hopkins University Press, 1985

Riese W: Galen on the Passions and Errors of the Soul. Translated by Harkins PW. Columbus, OH, Ohio State University Press, 1963

Rohde E: Psyche: The Cult of Souls and Belief in Immortality among the Greeks (1925). Translated from the 8th German edition by Hillis WB. London, 1950

Simon B: Mind and Madness in Ancient Greece: The Classical Roots of Modern Psychiatry. Ithaca, NY, Cornell University Press, 1978

Starobinski J: Trois Fureurs. Paris, Gallimard, 1974

Temkin O: The Falling Sickness, 2nd Edition. Baltimore, MD, Johns Hopkins University Press, 1971

Chapter 6

Stigma During the Medieval and Renaissance Periods

George Mora, M.D.

In this chapter the author traces the dual themes of the "good madman" and the "bad madman" in the history and literature of the Middle Ages and the Renaissance. Dr. Mora suggests that stigma was virtually unknown in the medieval attitude toward mentally ill persons because behavioral abnormalities were considered part of the divine plan for mankind. This tolerant view of mental illness continued into the Renaissance but began to wane when the theocentric view of the universe crumbled.

The Reformation brought a religious splitting of the Christian world, a disintegration of values, and a search for a scapegoat. The ensuing witch mania can be considered as an anticipation of the notion of stigma that would accompany mental illness from the rise of nationalism in the 17th century to our day.

Dr. Mora's scholarly analysis reminds us that the stigma associated with mental illness is inextricably connected to society's most fundamental beliefs. The study of history enables us to understand the emergence of contemporary attitudes.

Two points stand out in regard to mental illness in classical times: 1) mental illness was attributed to a disharmony among the various humors of the body, mainly to the overflow of the black bile (from which the term *melancholia* originated), leading to the belief that it had a somatic etiology (Klibansky et al. 1964); and 2) the notion of shame was present already in the Homeric poems, as a feeling justifying a variety of actions, many performed in a cruel way, aimed at redressing what was perceived as a damage to the status and the social role of the individual.

Thus, on the one side, mental illnesses, being undifferentiated from somatic illnesses, fell outside the boundaries of individual responsibility; on the other side, feelings related to shame were often projected in the realm of transcendental gods and goddesses, again relieving the individual from the responsibility for his or her actions (Dodds 1957; Snell 1953).

Such basic concepts, largely accepted by the early Roman culture, were later replaced by the emphasis on individual responsibility and, consequently, by the role attributed to passions in the Stoic philosophy (Pigeaud 1981; Roccatagliata 1986; Simon 1978). The early centuries of Christianity (used here in the broad sense of Judeo-Christian tradition) were characterized by a combination of the old naturalistic beliefs of mental illness as a somatic disease and the dimensions of the emotional life of the individual person. The novelty of the Christian message was that the ancient divinities, essentially a projection of human motives into the realm of the transcendental, were now replaced by the central figure of Jesus Christ, later followed by the mediating action of a succession of saints. The old therapeutic techniques of interpretation of dreams (Oppenheim 1956), incubation in the holy temples (Edelstein 1945; Meier 1967), and therapy of the word (Lain Entralgo 1970) continued in the new Christian version of supernatural visions, of extraordinary healing events taking place at shrines, and of pastoral counseling in the context of the sacraments of penance and repentance (Bonser 1963; Clebs and Jeakle 1964; Hamilton 1906; McNeil and Gamer 1965).

The theocentric perspective of Christianity encompassed the entire reality of the world, in which all beings, from the lowest to the highest, were viewed as an expression of God's theophany. From this viewpoint, all sorts of calamities, from the social (plague, famine, extenuating wars) to the individual (notably illness), were considered as an expression of God's inscrutable plans, as a form of punishment for human sinfulness and a test of endurance for mankind's lack of faith (Mora 1978, 1980). Such a theocentric perspective led to the conviction that events of any kind, from the most abject to the most sublime, were to be viewed as a manifestation of God's theophany, expressed through a hierarchy of progressively ascending degrees of perfection, from the lowest to the highest being (Lovejoy 1960).

Rather than a sign of stigma, the mentally ill were seen as living witnesses of the frailty of man, as prototypes of the lowest level of mankind, to be accepted as an intrinsic part of the great chain of beings. Instead of being hidden, they were to be exposed as examples of the frailty of man constantly at the mercy of the battle between the temptation of evil and the atonement achieved through grace.

Thus, on the one side stood the traditional picture of the wild man, as typified in the Biblical description of the king Nebuchadnezzar as a bad madman wandering throughout the country and presenting a dangerous, irresponsible, and animal-like type of behavior (Bernheimer 1952; Doob 1974). On the other side, in the chivalrous epic of the Middle Ages, stood, as a literary convention, the good madman as a transitional stage of the hero condemned to many trials and tribulations in order to finally obtain the hand of the beloved (Briffault 1965; Lowes 1914; Moore 1972; Nelli 1963; Scaglione 1963). Both prototypes, the "bad madman" and the "good madman," certainly appealed to the imagination of the static and largely illiterate society of the Middle Ages.

It would be difficult, if not impossible, to translate these behavioral characteristics of the madman into modern psychopathological concepts. What is certain is that evidence gathered through a variety of clues points to the existence of a certain percentage of mentally ill persons in the medieval society (Clarke 1975). The lack of a clear description of individual cases, compounded with the very likely high incidence of organic conditions— from avitaminosis, to malnutrition, infections, traumatic lesions, and other etiological factors—makes it very difficult to define the psychopathology affecting these individuals (Kroll 1973; Neugebauers 1978, 1979; Withwell 1936). Among the few exceptions are the chronicles of the lives of Charles VI, king of France, and of Henry VI, king of England (Autrand 1986; Brachet 1903; Dodu 1925; Ribadeau-Dumas 1969), as well as the report of abnormal behavior by a handful of artists and writers (Neaman 1975; Wittkower 1963). Very likely, in all these cases, the reason for preserving data on their mental condition was related to their unusual social status.

Most of the others presenting clear evidence of psychotic symptoms were left wandering in their own towns (a picture later typified in the Tom O'Bedlam vagrant) and accepted as natural members of the community, or kept at home under the supervision of members of the extended family or of neighbors. Undoubtedly, such supervision may have degenerated into cruel forms of restraint and abuse (Chaput 1975; Gilman 1982; Menard 1977; Rosen 1964). However, this has to be placed in the context of the feudal society of the time, in which the notion of individual freedom was virtually unknown and all kinds of severe punishments, up to death, inconceivable in our day, were daily occurrences, again as part of the overall divine plan. It is sufficient to say that suicide (a term that appeared only in the 18th century), rather than being viewed as the ultimate decision of the depressed person, was considered as despair ("desperatio") viewed as the outcome of a fight between virtues and vices that took place on the neutral background of the person (Bayet 1974; De Chapeaurouge 1960; Rosen 1971; Schmitt 1976).

The few mentally ill persons who were absolutely unmanageable and dangerous were turned over to the local authorities and thrown in dungeons and jails, at times for life. Only a relatively small number were cared for by religious orders in institutions that represented a combination of hospital, shelter, workshop, and penitentiary. (Interestingly, the word "penitentiary," then meaning a place to do penance for alleged sins, in time came to signify a prison for those convicted of crimes.) Some of these institutions were located in cities of central Europe, but, unfortunately, no record of individual inmates has been preserved (Desruelles and Bersot 1938; Jetter 1981; Leibbrand and Wettley 1961; Mora 1967; Panse 1964; Schipperges 1961).

The only exception is constituted by the 12th-century *Book of the Foundation,* dealing with cases of inmates at the St. Bartholomew's Church in Smithfield, London, in which, as expected, cases of apparent healing were attributed to supposed miracles performed by Bartholomew through visions and other supernatural means (Moore 1923; Wilmer and Scannon 1954). In the context of this heavily religious perspective, it is no wonder that a condition named *acedia* (literally, lack of spiritual zest), mainly affecting monks in isolation and characterized by a variety of symptoms from depression to obsessions, anxiety, and psychosomatic disorders, acquired importance as one of the seven deadly sins (Bloomfield 1952; Jackson 1981; Wenzel 1961). Indeed, this is an excellent example of the combination of psychological and religious factors in the etiology of mental illness. Much more dramatic, instead, were the cases of those who were allegedly possessed by the devil and who were exorcised through a complex, well-formulized ritual (Osterreich 1974).

In the light of all this, stigma was virtually unknown in the medieval attitude toward mentally ill persons, under the assumption that behavioral abnormalities were part of the divine plan for mankind. Understandably, contemporary historians have presented a view of the attitude toward persons with mental illness in the Middle Ages quite at variance from the traditional picture of the darkness of that period, or from the modern tendency to attach a stigma to mental illness. According to one (Bishop), "the insane were kindly treated, in general, and allowed to run at large or to dwell in almshouses without constraint unless they should be proved dangerous" (Bishop 1970); according to another (Neaman), although "the rural madman was a neglected and an often maltreated nomad . . . the medieval church may have been kinder to the madman than the seventeenth century hospital" (Neaman 1975). And for Huizinga, one of the most perceptive historians of our time, "on the one hand, the sick, the poor, the insane are objects of that deeply moved pity, born of a feeling of fraternity . . . , on the other hand, they are treated with incredible hardness and mocked" (Huizinga 1954).

The main theme briefly presented thus far in relation to the Middle Ages can be traced in the succeeding centuries of the Renaissance. As a matter of fact, continuity, rather than opposition, is the main trait that characterized those two periods. Of course, there were differences, too: the emergence of economic prosperity in many urban areas, of the nuclear family in which the woman played a significant role, of great creativity in arts and sciences, and, above all, of the awareness of the individuality of man, no longer perceived as an expression of God's theophany, but rather, as an image of the omnipotence of the Creator.

However, in opposition to this traditional optimistic view, recent historiography has pointed to the pessimistic view (i.e., the "dark side" of the Renaissance) (Battisti 1962; Haydn 1950; Kinsman 1974; Shumaker 1972; Yates 1979): the contrast between social classes, the widening gap between rulers and subjects, the tremendous impact of all sorts of calamities such as plague, the continuous threat posed by the Moslems, and the degeneration of the official Church leading to schisms and to religious wars. Hence, the Renaissance has been called an age of anxiety (Delumeau 1978): the security provided by the theocentric view of the universe was waning, while the rise of modern consciousness based on the interiority of moral values was not yet in sight.

All this created a situation of inner tension that led, on the one side, to a search for security from all sorts of occult, supernatural, or simply unusual beings and forces; while, on the other side, from a deeper perspective, to a satire of man trying to imitate God, best represented by Erasmus' *The Praise of Folly* (Erasmus 1979; Kaiser 1963; Screech 1980; Williams 1989) and by the phantasmagoric paintings of Bosch, Brueghel, and other artists of the Flemish school (Castelli 1952, 1953; Fierens 1947; Solier 1962). In all of them, there is a subtle interplay between salutary folly (i.e., true wisdom) and pure folly (i.e., deluded wisdom). The connection between the theme of folly as a literary and artistic convention and the theme of folly as insanity in the psychopathological sense has remained controversial to our day (Babb 1951; Bigeaud 1972; Feder 1980; Grassi and Lorch 1986; Lefebvre 1968; Lyons 1971).

The above-mentioned supernatural and unusual phenomena were expressed through interest in astrology, alchemy, and an array of other occult sciences, allegedly affecting human behavior by magically controlling unknown threatening forces and events. In the face of the all-encompassing insecurity and disintegration of values brought forward by the religious splitting of the Christian world at the time of the Reformation, a scapegoat had to be found to symbolically placate God's wrath and magically maintain that status quo so much sought by religious and secular leaders.

The image of the old woman, supposedly endowed with cryptic powers—going back to the traditional view of the woman as repository of the unexplainable phenomena of her monthly physiology and of the mysterious birth process, coupled with the traditional lore of the woman as repository of secret knowledge of herbs and other substances capable of healing, as well as of hurting (Forbes 1966; Michelet 1946; Mora 1984)—was considered to fit the prototype of the perverse power of the devil; the same devil which, in the preceding two centuries, had already been found to be at the basis of the heretical movements of the Albigenses, Cathars, and others. Slowly, the Inquisition came to equate heresy with sorcery and to subject both to the cruelest forms of punishment.

Understandably, the outbreak of the witch mania occurred especially in borderline areas of severe religious conflicts among Catholics and Protestants in France, Germany, and Switzerland, supported by some of the best theological, juridical, and political minds of the time. The matter of witchcraft mania, viewed in different keys—from the folkloristic to the religious—and in stringent contradiction with the recognition of the individuality and freedom of man and with the beginning of modern science, after the recent experience of the Holocaust, has received considerable attention from scholars of different disciplines. Increasingly, it is explained from the sociopsychological perspective as a magic attempt to counteract overwhelming feelings of anxiety toward the fear of annihilation through a symbolic sacrifice of the scapegoat (Russell 1987a, 1987b). From this viewpoint, the notion traditionally held in psychiatric circles—notably under the influence of Zilboorg (1941)—of alleged witches as being mentally ill, has been superseded by a widely accepted concept of these poor women as, instead, marginally existing individuals, cast in the role of witches by theologians supported by political authorities.

The *Malleus Maleficarum* (i.e., *Hammer for Witches*) (1486) by two German Dominicans, Heinrich Kramer and Jakob Sprenger, considered as a typical example of contemporary bigotry and superstition, continues to remain the worst document of misogyny ever published (Danet 1973; Kramer and Sprenger 1486/1971). Its value as an interesting report of psychopathological conditions, especially in terms of sexual aberrations—brought forward by the above-mentioned Zilboorg—is now placed in the wider perspective of sociopsychological deviance from current standards of acceptable behavior.

In the despotic climate of the Renaissance era, under the threat of the Inquisition, hardly anyone among the best minds of the time raised his voice against the horrors and the cruelties of the witchcraft mania, even in terms of the obvious absurdity of accepting at face value confessions obtained under torture. The few men who advanced new concepts on psychopathology and a humane stance toward mental illness (Vives) (Norena 1970; Vives 1917), or who took issue with some old concepts and cruel attitudes toward mentally ill persons (Paracelsus) (Mora 1967b; Paracelsus 1941), or who attempted to define insanity from the legal perspective (Zacchia) (Vallon and Genil-Perrin 1912; Zacchia 1635), shied away from taking a stand in regard to the persecution of witches. Only one of them, Johann Weyer (1563/1991), was effective, mainly in preventing some of these poor women from being tortured and executed; but his plea was so far ahead of his time that it did not become recognized until modern times.

All this may seem apparently peripheral to the issue of stigma toward mental illness; it acquires meaning, however, in considering that the unfavorable light cast on those poor women accused of witchcraft (some viewed as melancholic by the authors of the *Malleus Maleficarum* [1486/1971], as well as by Weyer) may indeed have represented a negative and condemning attitude toward mental illness. Perhaps it could be considered as an anticipation of the notion of stigma that would accompany mental illness from the rise of rationalism in the 17th century to our day.

Other expressions of the theme of folly, presenting grotesque and apparently irrational forms, came to be an intrinsic part of the culture. On the one side, there is evidence of the theme of folly in the gargoyles and other animal-like sculptures that are still visible in many cathedrals (Sheridan and Ross 1975; Valton 1915; Wildridge [nd]; Witkowski 1920). On the other side, at every important court, there was a jester, a dwarf or a midget, allegedly insane, but in reality allowed to mock, under facetious expressions, many aspects of the prevailing customs (Swain 1932; Welsford 1961). Finally, at a more popular level, the *"fête des fous,"* from which the modern carnival derived, provided an acceptable opportunity to express all kinds of instinctual urges suppressed by the official religiosity (Cox 1969).

For the more cultivated elite, the best representative examples of insanity, still in the framework of a literary convention, were provided by the hero's folly in Ariosto's *Orlando Furioso* (1502–1532) (Bonadeo 1970; Chesney 1977; DiTommaso 1973; Montano 1942) and in Cervantes' *Don Quixote* (1605–1615) (De Madariaga 1960; Gonthier 1962; Randall and Williams 1977). Naturally, any discussion on Renaissance psychopathology cannot omit even a cursory reference to Shakespeare's work. Like all his contemporaries, he was influenced by both the medical and the philosophical traditions of passions as strong human motives that can reach the level of illness. But his masterly description of passions, which has intrigued generations of scholars and, more recently, of psychiatrists and psychoanalysts, does not fit the cliché of insanity as traditionally held. True, the psychological conflicts portrayed in the Elizabethan dramas involve ethical and moralistic connotations as sources for moral instructions; but their protagonists, by not being considered insane, are not relevant to the notion of stigma (Babb 1951; Draper 1945).

More pertinent to our effort to detect the real contemporary attitudes toward mentally ill individuals in the Renaissance are the literary works that portrayed popular concepts of mental illness. In the book *The Hospital of the Incurable Fools* (1600) (Garzoni 1600; Laignel-Lavastine and Vinchon 1930; Padovani 1949) by the learned Italian monk Tommaso Garzone, a description is given of a series of abnormal individuals as seen by ordinary people, each one labeled with a particular adjective (e.g., odd, stubborn, extravagant). Although it is possible to identify in his descriptions modern psychopathological pictures, it is clear that the author's emphasis was on the nature, severity, and types of moral deviations from an ideal prototype of the normal individual.

In Thomas More's *Utopia* (1516), the fantastic description of an ideal society foretold the theme of social concern with, and rejection of, unacceptable misfortunes (Lameere 1963; More 1926, 1963). The same theme, viewed from the individual human perspective, was already anticipated in Sebastian Brant's poem *Ship of Fools* (1494) (Brandt 1962; Girard 1979; Maher 1982) and, a little later, in Hieronymus Bosch's painting of the same title (Boschere 1962; Combe 1957; Franger 1952; Tolnay 1966).

This artistic device of separating the fools from the rest of humanity may be viewed, as well, as an expression of the same trend that had already been carried on in reality, under religious auspices, in Spain (presumably on the wave of previous Arabic currents) in the early 15th century. There, in Valencia in 1409, a priest, Gilaberto Jofré, was so moved by a scene of mockery and sadism toward a mentally ill person by the populace in a street of the city as to inspire a number of outstanding citizens to open the first institution exclusively for the insane. His example was soon followed in other Spanish cities: Seville in 1436, Toledo in 1483, and Valladolid in 1489 (Bassoe 1945; Chamberlain 1962; Delgado Roig 1948; Dominguez 1967).

In the absence of reliable reports, it is impossible today to assess the condition of the inhabitants of these institutions. All that is known is that these places were staffed by religious orders with obviously great emphasis on respect for traditional values. Conversely, from a secular approach, a much more famous institution, the Hospital of St. Mary of Bethlehem in London, originally built as a shelter, progressively, in the 16th century, came to be used exclusively to lodge persons with mental illness. In this case, the scanty surviving records indicate that its main purpose was custody rather than care, and that by and large the inmates were subjected to all kinds of abuses and humiliations (Alleridge 1979; O'Donoghue 1914).

All this, in itself, points to a new attitude toward those affected by mental illness. It signifies the beginning of the trend toward the affirmation of individual guilt, forerunner of the moralistic emphasis of the Counter-Reformation and of the Baroque era. From then on, mental illness, coming to be recognized independently outside the realm of somatic illness—together with drunkenness, mental deficiency, delinquency, and other forms of aberrant behavior—would become the object of stigma by society, leading to what Foucault has called "the era of the great confinement" of the 17th century (Doerner 1981; Foucault 1965).

Everything thus far discussed, though understandable from the modern historiographical perspective, may appear rather remote from today's psychopathological concepts. Hence, it may be worth focusing on one well-documented example, the previously mentioned case of the insanity of King Charles VI of France. To make it more relevant to the issue of stigma, it may be useful to compare it with the case of insanity of George III, the last king of America. The choice was suggested by the circumstance that, exceptionally, for Charles VI, who lived between the late 14th and the early 15th centuries, his contemporary, Jean Froissart, left a vivid description of the king's life and mental illness in his *Chronicles,* which span between 1369 and 1410 (Froissart 1903, 1927–1928, 1929). For George III of England, a detailed description of his mental illness has been provided by Manfred Guttmacher, a well-known psychiatrist, in a comprehensive monograph (Guttmacher 1941, 1964). As a further rationale for the comparison, both kings appeared to have been affected by manic-depressive psychosis, although it has been submitted that George III may have suffered from porphyria, a point that has remained highly controversial (MacAlpine and Hunter 1969).

Charles VI's reign, which spanned between 1380 and 1422, was strained by all sorts of misfortunes: sickliness in his early childhood, opposition by his domineering uncles during the years of his minority, his absolute rule colored by a mixture of force and fear, the constant quarrels between the powerful lords (in particular between the Armagnacs and the Burgundys), the captivity of the popes in Avignon followed by the schism, the occupation of part of the French territory by the English during the Hundred Years War (1337–1453), the outbreak of plague, and, in the context of his immediate environment, duplicity and betrayals by the highest representatives of the nobility, the volatility and unfaithfulness of his queen consort, the tragic loss of two sons in their early twenties, and the emotional and unpredictable attitudes of the populace.

To follow Charles VI's mental condition, from his coronation at age 14, in 1390, to his death, on the background of such a complex scenario is certainly not easy, but Froissart's detailed report of the events helps to clarify at least some major points. The king suffered from intermittent episodes of depression and excitement, punctuated by long periods of inactivity followed by sudden outbursts, either belligerent, violent, revengeful, or grandiose. Some physicians were called, and they prescribed a regime of diet and rest that, of course, was not effective. Physical restraint was not part of the treatment, although it was applied at least once in an emergency situation.

The matter of his insanity was common knowledge. For the majority, his illness was inappropriate for a royal majesty; that is, it was a deviation from the orderly royal status and its supposedly inherent mental stability. Some clergymen, and some of his enemies, looked on his condition as a sort of punishment for his support of the anti-pope (Clement VII, 1378–1394) and for his sensual overindulgence. To appease the alleged wrath of God, one of his daughters was consecrated to the Virgin Mary and became a nun. In the superstitious and suspicious climate of the time, astrologists and cabalists were called in to determine whether evil powers, such as sorcery, had gained control of his mind, but no concrete evidence of this was found. Almost universally, the royal malady was considered God's will; that is, an example of God's inscrutable plans. Consequently, a number of masses, prayers, and processions were held to enhance his recovery. A wax figure in the shape of the king was sent to two religious places, both of which were known for the thaumaturgic powers of their respective saints. Not only was no particular stigma attached to his condition, which was largely viewed from the religious perspective, but, for the 42 years of his reign—during 30 of which he was insane—Charles VI was held by his subjects in constant pity and affection, and remained "Charles the Beloved" to the last.

The situation is entirely different in the case of George III, who suffered from five major attacks of mental illness between 1765 and 1810. Every possible means was employed by those close to him to keep his subjects from learning of his mental disorder, with the result that all sorts of rumors circulated about the royal malady. During the second attack of the disease in 1788, only reluctantly, by overcoming the opposition of the queen, was the Rev. Francis Willis, a physician known for his treatment of mental illness, entrusted with the care of the monarch. There was, in fact, concern that his particular area of specialty would indicate that his illustrious patient was afflicted with a mental condition. Such a condition followed a pattern of improvement and relapse. Later, Rev. Willis' services were no longer requested, as he was known to use his involvement with the royal family to boost his reputation. Another professional, Dr. Samuel Simon, a physician on the staff of St. Luke's Hospital and Bethlehem Hospital, was retained. But, in view of his specialty in mental disorders, his name was not included among those who signed the official bulletin. So, in conclusion, only after the king's death were frank disclosures of the real nature of his illness published.

These two different attitudes toward mental illness, that toward Charles VI in the Middle Ages and that toward George III in the Enlightenment, are so antithetical in regard to stigma that no further comment is necessary. Unfortunately, such a stigma is far from being overcome even today.

Conclusion

The Middle Ages and the Renaissance are, of course, gone forever, but a rethinking of them is far from being purely an antiquarian exercise. It would be naive, of course, to present an idealistic picture of the transcendental perspective of the Middle Ages or of the magic omnipotent perspective of the Renaissance. No matter how comprehensive of the entire reality of the world both perspectives were, each one had its "dark side." In the Middle Ages, although mentally ill persons may have been accepted with a great deal of tolerance, two other groups did not fit into the overall scheme of the great chain of beings: one was represented by the lepers (Brody 1974; Ell 1986; Richards 1977) and the other by the Jews (Cohen 1986; Marcus 1986;

Stow 1986). The difference between the two was obvious: in the first group, the "otherness" was patently manifested through physical ugly deformities; in the latter, the "otherness" was due to psychological, not visible, reasons. Both groups, thus, justified an attitude of stigma, no matter how much influenced by ambivalence: in the first instance, the interplay between human disgust and Christian pity; in the latter, the subtle, but no less pervasive feeling that Judaism was, indeed, the background from which Christianity sprang. Moreover, also not fitting into the great chain of beings, were, in a different way, two other groups: the heretics (Cullen 1985; Russell 1986) and the Moslems (Donner 1985). In the Renaissance, the witch, instead, superstitiously conceived as a repository of human calamities, became the prominent object of stigma. Thus, stigma existed in the Middle Ages as well as in the Renaissance, although it did not elicit guilt, for it was an intrinsic part of the prevailing Christian ideology rather than a matter of individual responsibility.

The Reformation, on the contrary, put the emphasis, in a dramatic way, on individual conscience and guilt. Later on, the Enlightenment, in a more subtle way, led to the secular ideals of universal equality and social concern for all. More recently, Western democratic postulates have unquestionably shown a tendency to spread all over, even to totalitarian regimes. In connection with this, a new awareness is emerging: that the immense issues facing today's world—from environmental pollution to population explosion and exhaustion of natural resources—can be addressed only from the global perspective.

Is it possible to advance anticipation on the future of the outcasts of society in the context of such a global perspective? Obviously, there is no easy answer to the overwhelming issues of the future of humanity. On a more modest scale, it is at least reassuring that human beings are progressively becoming *aware* (and this is no small achievement) of the issue of stigma and its negative connotations for society. Even assuming that stigma is intrinsic to human psychology, as an embodiment of the negative part of the self, such an awareness should lead to the hope that this time, in the context of secularism, mentally ill individuals will more readily become accepted and integrated into the community of mankind.

References

Alleride P: Management and mismanagement at Bedlam, 1547–1633, in Health, Medicine and Mortality in the Sixteenth Century. Edited by Webster C. Cambridge, UK, Cambridge University Press, 1979, pp 141–164

Alleride P: Bedlam: fact or fantasy? in The Anatomy of Madness: Essays in the History of Psychiatry, Vol 2. Edited by Bynum WF, Porter R, Shepherd M. London, Tavistock, 1985, pp 17–33

Autrand F: Charles VI: La folie du roi. Paris, Fayard, 1986

Babb L: The Elizabethan Malady: A Study of Melancholia in English Literature From 1580 to 1642. East Lansing, MI, Michigan State University Press, 1951 [reprinted 1965]

Bassoe P: Spain as the cradle of psychiatry. Am J Psychiatry 101:731–738, 1945

Battisti E: L'antirinascimento. Milano, Feltrinello, 1962

Bayet A: Le suicide et la morale (Paris, Alcan, 1922). New York, Arno, 1974

Bernheimer R: Wild Men in the Middle Ages: A Study in Art, Sentiment and Demonology. Cambridge, MA, Harvard University Press, 1952

Bigeaud M: La folie et les fous litteraires en Espagne, 1500–1650. Paris, Centre de Recherches Hispaniques, 1972

Bishop M: The Middle Ages. New York, American Heritage Press, 1970

Bloomfield M: The Seven Deadly Sins. East Lansing, MI, Michigan State University, 1952 [reprinted 1967]

Bonadeo A: Note sulla pazzia di Orlando. Forum Italicum 4:39–57, 1970

Bonser W: The Medical Background of Anglo-Saxon England: A Study in History, Psychology and Folklore. London, Wellcome Historical Medical Library, 1963

Boschere J de: Jerome Bosch et le fantastique. Paris, Albin Michel, 1962

Brachet A: Pathologie mentale des rois de France. Paris, Jachette, 1903

Brant S: The Ship of Fools (English translation). Translated by Zeydel E. New York, Columbia University Press, 1944. Reprinted New York, Dover, 1962 [Original edition: Basel, Der Narrenschiff, 1494]

Briffault RS: The Troubadours. Edited by Koons LF. Bloomington, IN, Indiana University Press, 1965

Brody SN: The Disease of the Soul: Leprosy in Medieval Literature. Ithaca, NY, Cornell University Press, 1974

Castelli E: Il demoniaco nell'arte. Milano, Electa, 1952

Castelli E (ed): L'umanesimo e il demoniaco nell'arte. Milano, Bocca, 1953

Castelli E (ed): L'umanesimo e la follia. Roma, Abete, 1971

Chamberlain AS: Early mental hospitals in Spain. Am J Psychiatry 123:143–149, 1966

Chaput B: La condition juridique et sociale de l'aliéné mental, in Aspects de la maraginalité au Moyen Age. Edited by Allard GH. Montreal, Les Éditions de l'Aurore, 1975, pp 38–47

Chesney E: The theme of folly in Rabelais and Ariosto. Journal of Medieval and Renaissance Studies 7:67–93, 1977

Clarke B: Mental Disorders in Early Britain. Cardiff, UK, University of Wales Press, 1975

Clebsch W, Jeakle C: Pastoral Care in Historical Perspective. Englewood Cliffs, NJ, Prentice-Hall, 1964

Cohen MA: Judaism in Southern Europe, in Encyclopedia of Religion, Vol 8. Edited by Eliade M. New York, Macmillan, 1986, pp 172–180

Combe J: Jerome Bosch. Paris, Tisne, 1957

Cox H: The Feast of Fools: A Theological Essay on Festivity and Fantasy. Cambridge, MA, Harvard University Press, 1969

Cullen B: Heresies, Western European, in Dictionary of the Middle Ages, Vol 6. Edited by Strayer JR. New York, Scribner's, 1985, pp 193–202

Danet A: Introduction, in Le marteau des sorciers (French translation). Translated by Danet A. Paris, Plon, 1973, pp 11–109

De Chapeaurouge D: Selbstmorddarstellungen des Mittelalters. Zeitschrift für Kunstwissenschaft 14:135-146, 1960

Delgado Roig J: Fundaciones psiquiatricas en Sevilla y nuevo mundo. Madrid, Paz Montalvo, 1948

Delumeau J: La peur en Occident, XIVᵉ-XVIIIᵉ siècles. Paris, Fayard, 1978

De Madariaga S: Don Quixote: An Introductory Essay in Psychology (English translation). Translated by De Madariaga S. New York, Oxford University Press, 1960

Desruelles M, Bersot H: L'assistance aux aliénés chez Arabes du VIIIᵉ au XIIᵉ siècles. Annales Medicopsychologiques 96:689-709, 1938

DiTommaso A: Insania and furor: a diagnostic note on Orlando's malady. Romance Notes 14:583-588, 1973

Dodds ER: The Greeks and the Irrational (Berkeley, CA, University of California Press, 1951). Boston, MA, Beacon Press, 1957

Dodu G: La folie de Charles VI. Revue Historique 150:161-188, 1925

Doerner K: Madmen and the Bourgeoisie: A Social History of Insanity and Psychiatry (English translation). Translated by Neugroschel J, Steinberg J. Oxford, UK, Blackwell, 1981

Dominquez EJ: The Hospital of Innocentes: human treatment of the mentally ill in Spain, 1409-1512. Bull Menninger Clin 31:285-295, 1967

Donner FD: Conquests of Islam, in Dictionary of the Middle Ages, Vol 6. Edited by Strayer JR. New York, Scribner's, 1985, pp 566-574

Doob P: Nebuchadnezzar's Children: Convention of Madness in Middle English Literature. New Haven, CT, Yale University Press, 1974

Draper JW: The Humors and Shakespeare's Characters. Durham, NC, University of North Carolina Press, 1945

Edelstein EJ, Edelstein L: Asclepius: A Collection and Interpretation of the Testimonies, 2 vols. Baltimore, MD, The Johns Hopkins University Press, 1945

Ell SR: Leprosy, in Dictionary of the Middle Ages, Vol 7. Edited by Strayer JR. New York, Scribner's, 1986, pp 549-552

Erasmus D: The Praise of Folly. Translated by Miller C. New Haven, CT, Yale University Press, 1979

Feder L: Madness in Literature. Princeton, NJ, Princeton University Press, 1980

Fierens F: Le fantastique dans l'art flamand. Bruxelles, Éditions du Circle d'Art, 1947

Forbes TR: The Midwife and the Witch. New Haven, CT, Yale University Press, 1966

Foucault M: Madness and Civilization: A History of Insanity in the Age of Reason. Translated by Howard R. New York, Random House, 1965 [Abridged edition of Histoire de la folie à l'âge classique. Paris, Plon, 1961]

Franger W: The Millenium of Hieronymous Bosch (English translation). Translated by Wilkins E, Kaiser E. London, Faber & Faber, 1952

Froissart J: The Cronycle of Syr John Froissart, 6 vols (English translation). Translated by Bouchier J. London, Nutt, 1903

Froissart J: Chronicles, 2 vols (English translation). Translated by Bouchier J. Oxford, UK, Blackwell, 1927-1928

Froissart J: Sir John Froissart's Chronicles of England, France, Spain . . . , 2 vols (English translation). Translated by Bouchier J. London, Smith, 1929

Garzoni T: The Hospital of Incurable Fools (English translation). Translated by

Nash T. London, Bollifant, 1600 [Original edition: L'hospedale de'pazzi incurabili. Ferrara, Cagnacini, 1586]

Gilman SL: Seeing the Insane. New York, Brunner/Mazel, 1982

Girard PF: La nef des fous et l'éloge de la folie: fiction litteraire et realité. Cahiers Medicaux 28:1915–1922, 1979

Gonthier DA: El drama psicologico del Quijote. Madrid, Studium, 1962

Grassi E, Lorch M: Folly and Insanity in Renaissance Literature. Binghamton, NY, Medieval and Renaissance Texts and Studies, 1986

Guttmacher MS: America's Last King: An Interpretation of the Madness of George III. New York, Scribner's, 1941

Guttmacher MS: The "insanity" of George III. Bull Menninger Clin 28:101–119, 1964

Hamilton M: Incubation or the Cure of Disease in Pagan Temples and Christian Churches. London, Simpkin, 1906

Haydn H: The Counter-Renaissance. New York, Harcourt, Brace & World, 1950

Huizinga J: The Waning of the Middle Ages (English translation). Translated by Middeleeuwen de H. Garden City, NY, Doubleday, 1954

Jackson S: Acedia: the sin and its relationship to sorrow and melancholia in medieval times. Bull Hist Med 55:172–185, 1981

Jetter D: Grundzüge der Geschichte das Irrenhauses. Darmstadt, Wissenschaftliche Buchgesellschaft, 1981

Kaiser W: Praisers of Folly: Erasmus, Rabelais, Shakespeare. Cambridge, MA, Harvard University Press, 1963

Kinsman RS (ed): The Darker Vision of the Renaissance. Berkeley, CA, University of California Press, 1974

Klibansky R, Panofsky E, Saxl F: Saturn and Melancholy. New York, Basic Books, 1964

Kramer H, Sprenger J: Malleus Maleficarum (1486) (English translation: London, Pushkin, 1948). Translated by Summers M. New York, Dover, 1971

Kroll JA: A reappraisal of psychiatry in the Middle Ages. Arch Gen Psychiatry 29:276–283, 1973

Laignel-Lavastine M, Vinchon J: La représentation symbolique des diverses formes da la folie: l'hôpital des fols incurables, in Les malades de l'esprit et leurs medecins du XVIᵉ au XIXᵉ siècle. Paris, Maloine, 1930, pp 87–100

Lain Entralgo P: The Therapy of the Word in Classical Antiquity (English translation). Translated by Rather LJ, Sharp JM. New Haven, CT, Yale University Press, 1970

Lameere J (ed): Les Utopies à la Renaissance. Bruxelles, Presses Universitaires de Bruxelles, 1963

Lefebvre J: Les foles et la folie: Étude sur les genres du comique et la création litteraire an Allemagne pendant la Renaissance. Paris, Klincksieck, 1968

Leibbrand W, Wettley A: Der Wahnsinn: Geschichte der abendlandischen Psychopathologie. Freiburg-München, Alber, 1961

Lovejoy AO: The Great Chain of Being: A Study of the History of an Idea (Cambridge, MA, Harvard University Press, 1936). New York, Harper, 1960

Lowes JL: The loverers maladyes of heroes. Modern Philology 11:491–546, 1914

Lyons BG: Voices of Melancholy: Studies in Literary Treatments of Melancholy in Renaissance England. London, Routledge & Kegan Paul, 1971

MacAlpine I, Hunter R: George III and the Mad-Business. London, Allen Lane, 1969

Maher WB, Maher B: The ships of fools: "Stultifera navis" or "Ignis fatuus." Am Psychol 37:756-761, 1982

Marcus IG: Judaism in Northern and Eastern Europe to 1500, in Encyclopedia of Religion, Vol 8. Edited by Eliade M. New York, Macmillan, 1986, pp 180-186

McNeil T, Gamer M (eds): Medieval Handbooks of Penance (New York, Columbia University Press, 1938). Reprinted New York, Octagon, 1965

Meier CA: Ancient Incubation and Modern Psychotherapy (English translation). Translated by Curtis M. Evanston, IL, Northwestern University Press, 1967

Menard P: Les fous dans la societé medievale. Romania 98:433-459, 1977

Michelet J: Satanism and Witchcraft: A Study in Medieval Superstition (English translation). Translated by Allison AR. New York, Citadel Press, 1946 [Original edition: La sorcière. Paris, Hachette, 1862]

Montano R: Follia e saggezza nel Furiosi e nell'elogio di Erasmo. Napoli, Guida, 1942

Moore JC: Love in Twelfth-Century France. Philadelphia, PA, University of Pennsylvania Press, 1972

Moore N: Book of the Foundations of St. Bartholomew's Church in London. London, Oxford University Press, 1923

Mora G: From demonology to narrenturm, in Historic Derivations of Modern Psychiatry. Edited by Galdston I. New York, McGraw-Hill, 1967a, pp 40-73

Mora G: Paracelsus' psychiatry: on the occasion of the 400th anniversary of his book "The Diseases That Deprive Man of His Reason." Am J Psychiatry 124:803-814, 1967b

Mora G: Mind-body concepts in the Middle Ages, I. J Hist Behav Sci 14:344-361, 1978

Mora G: Mind-body concepts in the Middle Ages, II. J Hist Behav Sci 16:58-72, 1980

Mora G: Witchcraft, heresy, and the scapegoat, in Evil, Self and Culture. Edited by Coleman Nelson M, Eigen M. New York, Human Sciences Press, 1984, pp 36-60

More T: Utopia. Translated by Campbell M. New York, Dutton, 1926

More T: The Complete Works of St. Thomas More, Vol 5. Edited by Carroll G, Murray J. New Haven, CT, Yale University Press, 1963

Neaman J: Suggestions of the Devil: The Origins of Madness. Garden City, NY, Anchor Books/Doubleday, 1975

Nelli R: L'érotique des troubadours. Toulouse, Privat, 1963

Neugebauers R: Treatment of the mentally ill and early modern England: a reappraisal. J Hist Behav Sci 14:158-169, 1978

Neugebauers R: Medieval and early modern theories of mental illness. Arch Gen Psychiatry 36:477-483, 1979

Noreña CG: Juan Luis Vives. The Hague, Martinus Nijhoff, 1970

O'Donoghue EG: The Story of Bethlehem Hospital From Its Foundation in 1247. London, Fisher Unwin, 1914

Oppenheim L: The interpretation of dreams in the ancient Near East. Transactions of the American Philosophical Society 46 (NS):179-373, 1956

Osterreich TK: Possession, Demoniacal and Other (English translation) (London, Kegan Paul, Trench, Trubner and Co, 1930). Translated by Ibberson D. New York, Causeway Books, 1974

Padovani G: "L'hospedale de'pazzi incurabili" di Tomaso Garzoni. Rassegna di Studi Psichiatrici 38:217–229, 1949

Panse F: Das psychiatrische Krankenhausewesen: Engwicklung, Stand, Reichweite und Zukunft. Stuttgart, Thieme, 1964

Paracelsus (Theophrastus von Hohenheim): The diseases that deprive man of his reason, in Four Treatises of Theophrastus von Hohenheim Called Paracelsus. Edited by Sigerist HE. Baltimore, MD, Johns Hopkins University Press, 1941, pp 129–212

Pigeaud J: La maladie de l'âme: Étude sur la relation de l'âme et du corps dans la tradition médico-philosophique antique. Paris, Les Belles Lettres, 1981

Randall D, Williams G (eds): Studies in the Continental Background of Renaissance English Literature. Durham, NC, Duke University Press, 1977, pp 186–201

Ribadeau Dumas, F: Madness in Power (English translation). Translated by Temperini KB. Philadelphia, PA, Chilton, 1969

Richards P: The Medieval Leper and His Northern Heirs. Totowa, NJ, Rowman and Littlefield, 1977

Roccatagliata G: A History of Ancient Psychiatry. Contributions in Medical Studies No 16. New York, Greenwood Press, 1986

Rosen G: The mentally ill and the community in Western and Central Europe during the late Middle Ages and the Renaissance. J Hist Med Allied Sci 19:377–388, 1964 [Reprinted in Rosen G: Madness in Society: Chapters in the Historical Sociology of Mental Illness. Chicago, IL, The University of Chicago Press, 1968]

Rosen G: History of the study of suicide. Psychol Med 1:267–285, 1971

Russell JE: Heresy: Christian concepts, in Encyclopedia of Religion, Vol 6. Edited by Eliade M. New York, Macmillan, 1986, pp 276–279

Russell JE: European witchcraft, in Dictionary of the Middle Ages, Vol 12. Edited by Strayer JR. New York, Scribner's, 1987a, pp 658–665

Russell JE: Witchcraft, in The Encyclopedia of Religion, Vol 15. Edited by Eliade M. New York, Macmillan, 1987b, pp 415–423

Scaglione A: Nature and Love in the Late Middle Ages. Berkeley, CA, University of California, 1964

Schipperges H: Der Narr und sein Humanum im islamischen Mittelater. Gesnerus 18:1–12, 1961

Schmitt JC: Le suicide au moyen âge. Annales Economies, Sociétés, Civilisations 31:3–38, 1976

Screech M: Erasmus and the Praise of Folly. London, Duckworth, 1980

Sheridan R, Ross A: Gargoyles and Grotesques: Paganism in the Medieval Church. Boston, MA, New York Graphic Society, 1975

Shumaker W: The Occult Sciences in the Renaissance. Berkeley, CA, University of California Press, 1972

Simon B: Mind and Madness in Ancient Greece: The Classical Roots of Modern Psychiatry. Ithaca, NY, Cornell University Press, 1978

Snell B: The Discovery of the Mind (English translation). Translated by Rosenmeyer TG. Cambridge, MA, Harvard University Press, 1953

Solier R: L'art fantastique. Paris, Albin Michel, 1962

Stow KR: Jews in Europe: after 900, in Dictionary of the Middle Ages, Vol 7. Edited by Strayer JR. New York, Scribner's, 1986, pp 86–94

Swain B: Fools and Folly During the Middle Ages and the Renaissance. New York, Columbia University Press, 1932

Tolnay C de: Hieronymus Bosch. New York, 1966

Ullersperger JB: La historia de la psicologia y de la psiquiatria en Espana (Spanish translation). Translated by Peset V. Madrid, Alhambra, 1954

Vallon C, Genil-Perrin G: La psychiatrie médico-legale dans l'oeuvre de Zacchia. Paris, Doin, 1912

Valton E: Les monstres dans l'art. Paris, Flammarion, 1915

Vives JL: Concerning the Relief of the Poor, or Concerning Human Need (English translation). Translated by Sherwood M. Studies in Social Work No 11. New York, New York School of Philanthropy, 1917

Welsford E: The Fool: His Social and Literary History (London, Faber & Faber, 1935). Garden City, NY, Doubleday, 1961

Wenzel S: The Sin of Sloth: Acedia in Medieval Thought and Literature. Chapel Hill, NC, University of North Carolina Press, 1961

Weyer J: Witches, Devils, and Doctors in the Renaissance [English translation of De praestigiis daemonum]. Edited by Mora G. Translated by Shea J. Binghamton, NY, Medieval and Renaissance Texts and Studies, 1991

Wildridge FT: The Grotesque in Church Art, 2nd Edition. London, Brown [nd]

Williams K (ed): Twentieth-Century Interpretations of the Praise of Folly. Englewood Cliffs, NJ, Prentice-Hall, 1969

Wilmer H, Scannon R: Neuropsychiatric patients reported cured at St. Bartholomew's Hospital in the twelfth century. J Nerv Ment Dis 119:1–22, 1954

Withwell JR: Historical Notes on Psychiatry. London, Lewis, 1936

Witkowski GJ: Les licenses dans l'art chrétien. Paris, Bibliothèque des Curieux, 1920

Wittkower R, Wittkower W: Born Under Saturn. New York, Random House, 1963

Yates F: The Occult Philosophy of the Elizabethan Age. London, Routledge & Kegan Paul, 1979

Zacchia P: Quaestiones medico-legales. Roma, 1621–1635

Zilboorg G: A History of Medical Psychology. New York, WW Norton, 1941

Chapter 7

The Devon Asylum: A Brief History of the Changing Concept of Mental Illness and Asylum Treatment

Louann Brizendine, M.D.

In this chapter Dr. Brizendine uses the history of the Devon Asylum to trace the changing concept of mental illness and treatment that emerged in the early 19th century. Advances in medical knowledge led to an advocacy of "moral treatment" and "non-restraint" and an interest in the patient's "total environment." Asylums developed as a response to these forces.

The vivid depiction of Dr. Bucknill, the director of the Devon Asylum, grappling with the issues of economics, administration, treatment methods, and overcrowding, gives life to the historical moment when the new specialty of psychiatry was developing. The treatment of mentally ill persons was becoming more humane in response to society's more humane views.

The medical knowledge of the late 18th and early 19th centuries in Britain, France, Germany, and America was in a transition that profoundly influenced the treatment of persons with mental illness. There was a growing acceptance among physicians and among laymen that the mind is a function of the brain and that mental physiology exists and is somehow related to "the mind" and therefore to behavior. The school of German somatic psychiatrists in the late 19th century eventually brought about the purest expression of this theory (Ackernecht 1968). The mechanical restraint and medical purges of the 18th century, which were applied in the well-known case of George III's mental illness, were to be replaced by "moral therapy" and "non-restraint." These were developed at the York Retreat by the Tukes, who came to doubt the efficacy of traditional "medical" remedies, not to mention the chains, whips, and other forms of physical restraint and coercion that were common "treatment" in that era. In America, Dr. Benjamin Rush was demanding that mental illness be freed from moral stigma and that the insane be treated with kindness under the supervision of physicians.

Developments in anatomy and physiology may have influenced the new notion of "partial insanity" elaborated by Pinel in France and some British authors. This was central to the new theory of "moral treatment" and "nonrestraint." If only a section and not the totality of a brain/mind was diseased, then an undamaged part of the brain was still left that could be reached by reason and the correct environment, the asylum, and that perhaps could help cure the damaged part of the brain.

The desired goal of therapy was to return the patient to control of himself or herself. This new therapeutic movement was optimistic about the curability of mental illness. The patient's "total environment" became such an important issue in restoring the patient's lost self-control in the early 19th century that writers on insanity devoted much discussion to asylum design.

The actual outcome of changing attitudes about mental illness can only be evaluated by a more detailed study of the individual asylums.

Communities in Britain were given permission by Parliament in 1828 to collect taxes for the express purpose of constructing a county asylum. The community of Devon and its asylum is an interesting and important case study. The system of treatment that evolved at the Devon County Asylum became a standard for psychiatrists mainly because of the work of its first medical superintendent, J. C. Bucknill (1817–1897). Bucknill was the founding editor of *The Asylum Journal* and author of the first modern text in psychiatry, entitled *A Manual of Psychological Medicine*. The Devon County Asylum was where he became experienced in treating mentally ill individuals. In this chapter I examine how the community of Devon viewed persons with mental illness, how they built the asylum, and how J. C. Bucknill treated cases of mental illness.

Establishment of the Devon Asylum

By 1844 the local authorities in Devon defined their view of the nature of insanity and the role of their asylum as follows: ". . . a lunatic asylum is more in the nature of a hospital than a prison; a place where curative treatment is applied to disease of a peculiar character and not a place of confinement or punishment" (Devon County *Minute Book* 1844). The Committee of local authorities hired a medical superintendent, J. C. Bucknill, and defined the asylum as a "hospital." This provides evidence that by 1844 the asylum authorities concurred with the new trend throughout the country of viewing insanity as a "disease."

For many years before 1844, complaint about vagrant mentally ill persons on the streets as well as the mentally ill individuals in the town workhouses had been plaguing the Devon County authorities (Devon County *Report of the Committee on the Proposed Lunatic Asylum* 1830). Because there was no county mental hospital, all that the county authorities could do for persons with mental illness was to send them off to a private "mad house." The type of treatment was quite likely to be chains, whips, or medical purges. The town or parish, not the county, was responsible for payment, possibly for the rest of the person's life. Thus this was an unpopular arrangement for the towns. It was cheaper to keep mentally ill persons in the town workhouses than to build an asylum.

The county magistrates first proposed building a county mental hospital in Devon at the quarterly meeting in July 1829 (*Exeter Flying Post*, July 16, 1829, p. 3). An example of the sentiment expressed at this meeting was that of the Rev. Palmer, Vicar of Yarcombe, who raised the issue of "what the county should do to care properly for the mentally ill." He was not alone in his concern. Another magistrate spoke at the same meeting, saying, "Something ought to be done for these wretched objects who, whilst remaining in their communities[,] are too generally doomed to spend their days in wretchedness . . . and will remain the sport and byword of the idle, the terror of the timid, and cut off from all hope of cure" (*Exeter Flying Post*, July 16, 1829, p. 3). Public abuse of mentally ill individuals did concern the county magistrates. It appears that they were also aware that better treatment and even cure was possible "nowadays." A subcommittee, led by Rev. Palmer, was appointed to study the numbers of persons with mental illness and how other counties had gone about building their asylums.

At the next quarterly meeting, Rev. Palmer's subcommittee announced that it had counted 195 poor mentally ill persons residing in the county of Devon. The subcommittee estimated that a county hospital could be built for a considerable amount of money. Although there was no disagreement about the need, there was considerable disagreement about the cost. The community newspaper, *The Exeter Flying Post*, reported these meetings to the public. It announced the intention of the county to build the hospital and its probable cost. Within a week the public responded angrily with 18 petitions to the county magistrates against the asylum, stating, for example, that the asylum "is inexpedient and unnecessary since the poor houses and workhouses are good enough" (*Exeter Flying Post*, April 22, 1830, p. 3). What was the explanation for such strong local opposition? These petitions seem to go against the public trend that was expressed in the national reform movement.

On examination of the local documents, several major issues stand out, the first of which may explain the petitions from the towns. Until this time, town authorities had complete control over the placement of their mentally ill citizens. Each workhouse received money for keeping a mentally ill person. It was discovered that many of the petitions had actually been falsified by the authorities of several workhouses (*Exeter Flying Post*, October 21, 1835, p. 3). Financial opposition was not only from the taxpayers but also from the workhouses who stood to lose income.

The second issue is that the year of 1830 marked the beginning of an economic recession throughout Britain, especially for agricultural regions like Devon. During the economic recession support for mentally ill individuals was kept alive, at least on the national level and in the press. In London, Lord Ashley was in charge of the Parliamentary Select Committee on the Mentally Ill. He continued to make mental illness his cause célèbre both in Parliament and in the press. From 1832 to 1840 four major bills dealing with reform for the treatment of persons with mental illness passed. In 1834 Parliament passed a law *requiring* town authorities to take responsibility for finding and paying for a "proper place within 14 days" for any person with mental illness found in their workhouse (Poor Law Amendment Act 1834).

In 1835 local support for the asylum increased by the appointment of a new chairman to the Board of Magistrates in Devon: the influential Earl of Devon, a long-time friend of the local reformer Rev. Palmer. In the first meeting he made a motion that "a more effectual provision should be made in our county for the care and maintenance of the indigent mentally ill" (*Exeter Flying Post*, July 2, 1835, p. 3). As a concession to the town authorities, the county magistrates guaranteed voting rights for the towns on all issues concerning the county hospital and its patients (*Exeter Flying Post*, April 6, 1837, p. 3). So after 6 years of conflict the county asylum had finally been funded in 1837.

The Devon authorities now needed to construct and develop an asylum. The governing bodies of other counties with asylums provided no consistent precedent. The County of Devon surely knew about the miserable experience of its neighboring county, Cornwall. The authorities there had hired a nonmedical superintendent who had not provided for the medical needs of the patients, resulting in several fatalities (Cornwall County *Minute Book of the Cornwall Asylum* 1828). But there were also counties that had no problems with laypersons as superintendents. Devon was very cautious. It decided to hire a medical man and preferably one with experience in treating mental illness (Devon County *The Minute Book of the Committee of Visitors* 1841–1856). Finding such a person was not easy, because well-trained medical doctors who had experience and interest in treating mental disease had just recently come to the forefront (Conolly 1832). Young physicians had become increasingly interested in mental disease. A group of medical superintendents of mental hospitals had just formed an association that was the forerunner of the Royal Medical Psychiatric Association. One of its members, Dr. Sutherland, captured the attitude of the day: "The subject of [mental illness] has been growing in importance ... and is no longer seen as something supernatural ... nor degraded as followed by men of mere trade, but men have arisen of late years who have studied it as a science and have elevated it to the rank which it ought to hold in medicine" (*The Asylum Journal* 1855).

In 1844 Devon selected Dr. J. C. Bucknill from 54 applicants. Bucknill had graduated first in his class in medical school and then studied surgery under Listor for a year before opening a medical practice in Chelsea. He was from a medical family consisting of both surgeons and medical men. As a young physician Bucknill's enthusiasm for mental science developed in the atmosphere of new discovery. He was truly one of the new generation of mental physicians. Devon had made a fortunate choice: not only was Bucknill to become one of the most respected psychiatrists of his day, both in Britain and in America, but he was involved in every aspect of running the asylum. The type of treatment for mentally ill persons at Devon became well known as a standard through his writings.

The asylum was partially staffed 2 months before the first patient was admitted. In the surrounding town, 10% to 15% of the population are listed as having sought employment at the asylum (*Exminister Register of Baptisms* 1845–1901). The first patients were admitted in August 1845, and 18 months later the asylum census was 244.

Treatment at the Asylum

It was not common practice in most asylums to keep detailed written reports on patients. However, Devon Asylum was an exception. Dr. Bucknill did in fact keep records on a few patients. Before the asylum opened he organized his casebooks into two columns: 1) "Symptoms When Admitted," and 2) "Progress of Case After Admission."

The first recorded case history is a 17-year-old lace maker admitted from the local workhouse on August 2, 1845. The alledged cause of insanity was "moral." In the history she was said to have been "low spirited" for 8 to 9 months prior to admission because her lover had deserted her. The parents were questioned as to whether the lover may have given her "noxious drugs" or physically injured her. Her mother revealed that the girl had gone through periods of intense "exertion" and "had been much depressed" at other times in her life from age 12 years on, not just recently. It was recorded that she had no delusions, never tried violence against herself or others, and was worse during the full moon. There was some allusion to hereditary predisposition; the first sentence that Bucknill wrote on the case was, "Always very nervous, like her father who was about 50 when she was born."

Under "general state of mind," her senses were noted to be unimpaired, but she was silent, often laughed, and sung tunes without words, and seemed very happy. Her "propensities" were recorded as "sometimes wet, but not dirty." The notes stated that her "attitude and locomotion" were "bizarre posturing" and that she "places herself in extraordinary positions in the corners, etc., puts her head down, seems disinclined to walk about and will not take food without being forced." This case was one of Bucknill's early successes, for she was discharged 11 months later and recorded as "recovered" (*Medical Casebook*, Patient Number 37).

Other patients were not so fortunate. Often the workhouses sent to the asylum their elderly, eccentric, infirm patients who could no longer work. These patients arrived in terrible physical condition, and all Bucknill could do was to watch them die. For example, a 50- to 60-year-old female was admitted on August 7, 1845, whose alleged cause of insanity of 3 years' duration was "moral and physical." She expired the same day of "old age and bronchitis" (*Medical Casebook*, Patient Number 55).

The majority of patients admitted neither died nor recovered during that first year. Over 70% of the patients who were admitted that first year were still confined after 18 months. An example of this kind of patient is a 28-year-old female admitted on August 28, 1845, whose alleged cause of insanity was "moral." At the time of admission the duration of her illness was recorded as "four years." There are no other entries on the page until August 24, 1872, where it is recorded she died of "severe Diarrhea."

The most frequently recorded "alledged cause of insanity" was "moral." What distinguished a moral case from any other case of insanity? If an event in a patient's life could be pointed to as the inciting event, then Bucknill categorized this as "moral." Until March 1846, Bucknill made no entries under "general treatment." After 1846, most patients whose cases Bucknill recorded were given some medicinal remedy, although it is not clear from the records how frequently the remedy was given. Many patients were given "warm baths" and "light shower baths." "Opium" and "leeches" as well as "purges" seemed to have been used often. Only a few patients have any notes under "Progress of Case After Admission." For one patient, for whom there was an assessment 18 months after his admission, it is noted that "there is no appreciable change with this patient, his mind is still filled with delusions, some of his old ones he has laid aside, others he retains" (*Medical Casebook*, Patient Number 55).

The initial paragraph of Bucknill's annual report always summarized the numbers of patients admitted or discharged and the number of patients who had died. He then subdivided the number discharged into those who left cured, improved, or unimproved. In the year 1847 he discharged 30 patients "cured," 2 "improved," and 1 "unimproved" (Devon County *Annual Report to the Committee* 1848, p. 7). Later in the same report he stated his belief that the following system of treatment, although difficult, would increase the cure rate for the next year:

Occupation of the mind and body by exercise and recreation, which is so essential to the rational treatment of the insane ... Amusements required to be diversified; the use of books to be directed and encouraged: And the mind, preoccupied by delusion and by egotism, needs to have more wholesome food for reflection pressed upon it. Industrial occupations are of utmost service ... the exercise of music ... and the practice of the attendant and better educated patients reading aloud ... during the ensuing year we hope to make further efforts in this direction believing the cure of many patients may be expedited thereby. (Devon County *Annual Report to the Committee* 1848, p. 9)

The following year the number of patients he discharged as "cured" increased to 42. He considered this a marked improvement over the previous year's and calculated the percentage cured as 36.2% by comparing the number of patients cured to the number of admissions.

In 1849 there were no rates reported because of a cholera epidemic that swept through the Asylum killing over 60% of the patients. By the 1850 report the cure rate was even better, but a change in category occurred. The number "cured" was no longer reported, but "cured and recovered" were now lumped together. Whether this was an intentional or an unintentional way of improving the "cure" rate is unclear.

Cures, recoveries, and discharges were not the singular concern of the Administrative Committee at the Asylum, however. The focus of the Committee was how to require the Poor Law Guardians to send their mentally ill residents to the Asylum at the earliest possible date. This is not to say that concern for the cure and recovery of patients did not exist, but in the words of the Committee: "Your Committee beg leave to remark that the value of the Asylum ought not to be measured only by the number of patients who have been cured. To these helpless objects the Asylum affords freedom from annoyance, cleanliness, warmth, food and clothing ... and each of them receives such general and medical treatment as the peculiarities of the case requires" (Devon County *Annual Report to the Committee* 1848, p. 5). The enthusiasm over their humanitarian accomplishment was still high and had not yet been ruined by the problems of a low cure rate and subsequent overcrowding.

Explanations for the low cure rate were twofold. First, patients had not been sent in soon enough by the Poor Law Guardians to the Asylum for proper care, thereby allowing the chronicity of the illness to become fixed. This delay was blamed on the reluctance of the Poor Law Guardians to send the patients to the Asylum for financial reasons. Second, a "proper environment" for cure could not be maintained in an overcrowded asylum with terminal, medically ill patients. After 1850, this latter reason was quoted more and more frequently.

Overcrowding in Devon Asylum started in 1849, 4 years after its opening. The Asylum was built for a census of 400, and in 1850 the census was 412.

County asylums could not refuse patients who had been "certified" by the requisite medical authority. Many terminally ill patients were ridded from workhouses by sending them to the Asylum. But discharge from the Asylum of "docile, chronic patients" was resisted by Dr. Bucknill, based on the "fear of dangerousness" outside the asylum environment. On the other hand, Dr. Bucknill did not want to close the doors to admission for fear that the young, first-episode "curables" would not be sent in quickly enough and thereby become incurable.

The payment rate for patients had been decreasing. In 1844 it was 10 shillings per patient, and by 1850 it was 7.6 shillings per patient. As the number of patients increased, the cost per patient decreased, so there was little incentive on the part of the community to reduce numbers at the Asylum. This financial aspect of overcrowding was pleasing to both the county and the town authorities.

By 1850, the patient census and the cost effectiveness of numbers were major issues for the Committee of Visitors. In November 1850, Bucknill had declared the female wards to be over capacity, and the male wards followed this trend, becoming over capacity by October 1851. The new era of overcrowding had begun. The Committee and the Guardians did not work together to help reduce the overcrowding but continued to argue for years over sending terminally ill patients to the Asylum and demanding the discharge of chronic patients from the Asylum. The town was tired of paying for them. The situation was not unique to Devon, nor England. In subsequent years, overcrowding was to become the Waterloo of the asylum system.

Dr. Bucknill, the Asylum System, and the Profession of Psychiatry

The treatment of patients at the Devon Asylum, as well as the problems of overcrowding, became well known through the writings of Dr. Bucknill. He also was instrumental in developing the profession of psychiatry around the asylum system of treatment. This new medical subspecialty's first professional organization, founded in 1841, was called "The Association of Medical Officers of Lunatic Asylums." The organization's title was soon changed to "The Association of Medical Officers of Hospitals for the Insane." This change in title reveals two concerns of the new group. First, the association was concerned with standardizing and modernizing terminology, using "insane" instead of "lunatic," and second, the members saw themselves as medical doctors who treated sick people in a "hospital," not a "mad house." Membership was restricted to medical officers of hospitals and asylums for the insane and qualified medical men who treated insanity. The members were reportedly anxious to compare notes on the various practical issues of treatment (*The Asylum Journal* 1854). It was in this spirit of a common endeavor that the members agreed to record the "medical" and "moral" treatment in use at each hospital. An attempt to be scientific in the statistical sense was made by agreeing to use uniform registers and tabular statements in the annual report of each hospital for easy comparison (*The Asylum Journal* 1854, p. 15). Some of the early papers read at meetings were on reporting statistical observations, methods of recording "morbid appearances" of the insane, asylum construction, and "homicidal mania." Reports on current medical therapeutics were read, and individuals with pathological conditions were sometimes exhibited.

The *Asylum Journal* became the written forum for the new psychiatric profession. It established the first guidelines for acceptable standards of psychiatric practice; it contained statistics on all the asylums so that comparisons could be made; and it provided a mechanism for giving feedback to Parliament and local government. Bucknill, as the editor, strongly influenced the direction of the early profession. He not only selected the articles that would appear but also wrote much of the first seven volumes (Bucknill and Tuke 1858). He saw *The Journal* as psychiatry's mouthpiece to the public as well as to the profession. As Bucknill wrote,

> Publicity in matters affecting the welfare of the insane poor is much needed. Publicity which, without delay, may inform all who are entrusted with the care of the insane of the most recent amelioration in their treatment and thus remove from abuses as they arise and prevent their growth and continuance. A publicity which can only be secured by a journal devoted to the purpose and aided by the adherence to the new system throughout the Kingdom. (*The Asylum Journal* 1854, p. 11)

The *Journal* served as a monitor for the activities of those groups who controlled the implementation of lunacy reform. Bucknill also saw it as a platform to educate the Commissioners in Lunacy who, he said, "lacked an understanding of the first great principle of insanity: that insanity is a curable state of bodily and brain disease" (*Journal of Mental Science* 1858, 4:51).

Through *The Asylum Journal* the "non-restraint method" of treatment became the battle cry of psychiatrists who were members of the Association.

Those psychiatrists who continued to use mechanical restraints on patients were ostracized in various ways by the new professional association. As Bucknill wrote in *The Journal*:

> "Physicians who treat insanity with penal remedies are not likely to regard its causes as a pathological condition of the organism ... but those who regard it as a fermentation of the spiritual essence ... easily and logically persuade themselves that sharp penal remedies are useful and justifiable in its treatment." (*Journal of Mental Science* 1858)

Conclusion

Did the treatment of patients by Dr. Bucknill at Devon Asylum live up to his written word? Although existing records are somewhat sparse, it appears that Bucknill used mechanical restraints only once to keep a patient from scratching herself. "Seclusion" and "shower baths" were often used in response to a patient "hitting Dr. Bucknill" or a staff member (*The Annual Report of the Committee* 1847–1850). There is evidence that he did examine some brains postmortem (*Casebooks* 1845). The existing casebooks are well organized, but his notes on most patients are sparse at best. Usually, the patient's name, date of admission, and date of death or discharge were the only entries he made in the huge 24-inch by 18-inch casebook (*Casebooks* 1845). Having 400 patients to care for and an asylum to administer, not to mention his prolific writing, may have left Bucknill little time to treat patients or to record observations.

The issue of "non-restraint" was more of a rallying point than a method of treatment. "Moral" therapy was the concept of total treatment that reflected society's changed view of the stigma of mental illness. A careful look at individual asylums like Devon allows us to look at the local reality of the implementation of reform. The new subspecialty of psychiatry, which grew up around the asylum system, was equally enthusiastic about cure in the beginning; however, as overcrowding increasingly became a problem, psychiatrists' attention turned more and more to administration.

The enthusiasm of the reform movement, propelled by the social times and economic realities of the changing structure of Industrial England, opened the way for actual change not only in reducing the stigma of mental illness but also in improving treatment in asylums. However, as mentioned above, overcrowding, in part due to unbridled enthusiasm, was the Waterloo of the asylum system. Perhaps even an overcrowded asylum was an improvement over the previous standard of care in workhouses and many "mad houses." Certainly society's view of mentally ill persons had changed, and, consequently, the treatment of this group had become more humane.

References

Ackernecht EH: A Short History of Psychiatry, 2nd Ed. New York, Hafner, 1968

Bucknill JC, Tuke D: A Manual of Psychological Medicine (1858). New York, Hafner Publishing, 1968 [A facsimile of the 1858 edition]

Conolly J: Four Lectures on the Study and Practice of Medicine. London, Sherwood, 1832

Unpublished Primary Source Material

Cornwall County: Minute Book of the Cornwall Asylum, 1828. Unpublished document, Cornwall County Record Office.

Devon County: Annual Report of the Committee of Visitors, Devon County Quarter Sessions 1847-1850 and 1854-1868. Unpublished reports, Devon County Record Office, Exeter, UK

Devon County: Annual Report of the Medical Superintendent of the Devon County Lunatic Asylum, Devon County Quarter Sessions 1848-1850 and 1854-1865. Unpublished reports, Devon County Record Office, Exeter, UK

Devon County: Medical Casebooks from Devon Asylum. Unpublished documents, Devon County Record Office, Exeter, UK

Devon County: Minute Book of the Committee of Visitors of Pauper Lunatics at Devon County Asylum, 1841-1856. Unpublished document, Devon County Record Office, Exeter, UK

Devon County: Report of the Committee on the Proposed Lunatic Asylum, Devon County Quarter Session, Midsummer 1830. Unpublished report, Devon County Record Office, Exeter, UK

Further Reading

Articles

Bynum WF: Rationales for therapy in British psychiatry, 1780-1835. Med Hist 18:317-334, 1974

Jones K: Society looks at the psychiatrist. Br J Psychiatry 132:321-332, 1978

McCandless P: Build! Build! The controversy over the care of the chronically insane in England, 1855-1870. Bull Hist Med 53:553-574, 1979

Patch IL: Treatment or punishment? A 19th-century scandal. Psychol Med 6:143-149, 1976

Scull AT: Moral treatment reconsidered: some sociological comments on an episode in the history of British psychiatry. Psychol Med 9:421-428, 1979

Books

Barton W: The History and Influence of the American Psychiatric Association. Washington, DC, American Psychiatric Press, 1987

Becher Rev JT: An Address to the Public on the Nature, Design and Constitution of the General Lunatic Asylum Near Nottingham. Newark, UK, Ridge, 1811

Browne WAF: What Asylums Were, Are and Ought to Be. London, 1837

Bucknill JC: Unsoundness of Mind in Relation to Criminal Acts. London, 1854

Bucknill JC: The Psychology of Shakespeare. London, 1859

Bucknill JC: The Mad Folk of Shakespeare. London, 1867

Burnett CM: Insanity Tested by Science. London, 1852

Burton R: Anatomy of Melancholy (1621). Edited by Floyd Dell. New York, Tudor Publishing, 1927

Busfield J: Managing Madness: Changing Ideas and Practice. London, Hutchinson Press, 1986

Castel R: The Regulation of Madness. Translated by Halls WD. London, Polity Press, 1988

Clark B: Mental Disorder in Earlier Britain. Cardiff, University of Wales Press, 1975

Conolly J: Treatment of the Insane Without Mechanical Restraint. London, 1856
Conolly J: An Inquiry Concerning the Indications of Insanity. London, Sherwood, 1830
Digby A: Madness, Morality and Medicine: A Study of the York Retreat, 1796–1914. Cambridge, UK, Cambridge University Press, 1985
Gill GN: The Prevention and Cure of Insanity. London, 1814
Granville M: The Care and Cure of the Insane: Report of Lancet Commission, Vols I and II. London, 1877
Grob G: The State and the Mentally Ill. Chapel Hill, NC, University of North Carolina Press, 1966
Grob G: Mental Institutions in America: Social Policy to 1875. New York, Free Press, 1973
Grob G: Mental Illness and American Society, 1875–1940. Princeton, NJ, Princeton University Press, 1983
Grob G: The Inner World of American Psychiatry, 1890–1940. New Brunswick, NJ, Rutgers University Press, 1985
Hill RG: Total Abolition of Personal Restraint in the Management of Lunatic Asylums. London, 1839
Hunter R, Macalpine I: Three Hundred Years of Psychiatry: 1535–1860. London, Oxford University Press, 1963
Hunter R, Macalpine I: Psychiatry for the Poor. London, Oxford University Press, 1974
Jones K: Mental Health and Social Policy, 1845–1959. London, Routledge & Kegan Paul, 1955
Leigh D: The Historical Development of British Psychiatry. New York, Pergamon, 1961
MacGregor AJ: Historical Landmarks in the Treatment of Insanity. London, 1894
Mercier C: Lunatic Asylums: Their Organization and Management. London, 1894
Parry-Jones W: The Trade in Lunacy. London, 1972
Peterson JM: The Medical Profession in Mid-Victorian London. Berkeley, CA, University of California Press, 1978
Porter R: A Social History of Madness. New York, Weidefeld and Nicholson, 1988
Porter R: Mind-Forged Manacles. Cambridge, MA, Harvard University Press, 1987
Prichard JC: A Treatise on Insanity. London, 1835
Ramon S: Psychiatry in Britain: Meaning and Policy. London, Croom Helm Press, 1985
Riese W (ed): Historical Explorations in Medicine and Psychiatry. New York, 1978
Rosen G: Madness in Society. Chicago, IL, University of Chicago Press, 1968
Rothman D: The Discovery of the Asylum. Boston, MA, 1971
Skultans V: Madness and Morals: Ideas on Insanity in the 19th Century. London, Routledge & Kegan Paul, 1975
Sutton SB: Crossroads in Psychiatry: A History of the McLean Hospital. Washington, DC, American Psychiatric Press, 1986
Thurman J: Statistics of Insanity. London, 1841
Tomes N: A Generous Confidence. Cambridge, UK, Cambridge University Press, 1984
Tuke DH: Reform in the Treatment of the Insane. London, 1832
Tuke DH: Chapters in the History of the Insane. London, 1882
Tuke S: Description of the Retreat. Philadelphia, PA, 1813

Verwey G: Psychiatry in an Anthropological and Biomedical Context. Amsterdam, Reidel Publishing, 1985

Young RM: Mind, Brain and Adaptation in the 19th Century. Oxford, UK, Oxford University Press, 1970

Chapter 8

Madness and the Stigma of Sin in American Christianity

Norman Dain, Ph.D.

In this chapter Dr. Dain explores the attitudes toward mental illness that are expressed by a variety of Christian groups. He examines the work of Jonathan Edwards and Cotton Mather during the Great Awakening of the 18th century. He then moves on to consider both liberal and fundamentalist strains in the 19th and 20th centuries. He concludes that Christianity has a basic problem with associating mental illness with sin, a problem that in practical terms has been resolved "by rendering the afflicted unto Caesar."

The traditional belief among Christians that madness is often a punishment "visited by God on the sinner" (Neaman 1975) predominated in American society during the 17th century and remained quite influential thereafter. Insofar as traditional Christianity stresses sin as the cause of insanity, although by no means the only cause, persons with mental illness become stigmatized. Of course, all forms of misfortune, including so-called physical illnesses, were also often considered the wages of sin. But illnesses that were considered physical, with the notable exceptions of venereal diseases and alcoholism, were, especially from the 18th century onward, perceived to have somatic causes that increasingly were not considered to involve sin. It is true that somatic or natural causes in the 18th and early 19th centuries were often viewed as God working through nature, so that in theory physical illness was no less God's punishment for sin than were diseases caused by the direct intervention of God or the devil by miraculous means. In practice, however, leading religionists, influenced by the rationalism of the Enlightenment and by modern science, came to accept most physical disease as not commonly the consequence of sin, an attitude increasingly shared by the general population and one that supported the construction of mental hospitals as the best places to treat the so-called "insane." Even when responsibility for disease was attributed to the victim's action or inaction, such behavior was regarded not as sinful but as ignorant or careless.

Many religious people and clergymen subscribed to the physician's view that although personal behavior could cause disease or at least contribute to its onset—for example, poor diet, lack of exercise, bad work habits, or tobacco smoking—such behavior did not constitute an act against God and therefore was not sinful. And of course the Society of Friends, an evangelical sect, not only took a benevolent attitude toward mentally ill persons but also founded mental hospitals in both England and America; Quakers were leaders in the movement for humane care of the disabled and deviant.

But those of the religious who stressed the Bible as the literal source for understanding insanity were more likely to see that disorder as the consequence of personal sin. Asked what sins a madman or his parents had committed, Jesus said that neither the sick man nor his parents had sinned; although Jesus practiced exorcism in the New Testament, it seems that he believed that mental illness was sometimes unrelated to sin. Still, many of the clergy and the public had almost from the first considered most, if not all, cases of insanity as punishment for sin. After all, insane persons did at times curse God, engage in immoral sexual relations, and even commit murder. This traditional view of madness as the wages of sin was reinforced in the religious struggles after the Protestant Reformation. Once England officially became a Protestant nation, 17th-century Protestants and Catholics competed to show their respective ability to cure the possessed. Catholics secretly and not so secretly practiced exorcism; Protestants, pressed to respond with similar apparently effective means of restoring the afflicted, prayed and fasted. To both sides, affirming the supernatural nature of possession and then possession itself as a contest between good and evil, God and the devil, confirmed the validity of Christianity; successful exorcism or prayer and fasting certified Catholicism or Protestantism as "true" Christianity. The poor victim in any case retained the stigma of sin.

The Protestant religious in what is now the United States included many Calvinists who believed that insanity was derived from sin. Although early American Protestants did not need to worry overmuch about competition with Catholics over possession and exorcism, various disputes among Protestants led to competition that involved insane persons as unwitting pawns. The growth of religious liberalism and secularism in the 18th century met resistance most notably in the Great Awakening that in the 1730s and 1740s split Calvinist and other established churches into warring factions. In this process evangelicals often adopted the more conservative negative attitude toward insane individuals. It should be noted, however, that the central issue for those who saw insanity as sinful was not so much the nature of insanity but the preservation of the biblical view of the subject: to reject the role of sin in the etiology of madness was equivalent to rejecting the Bible as the ultimate and inerrant source for Christian beliefs. The concern of revivalists then, and subsequently, was usually not so much with insanity as with defending their conception of Christianity against modernist liberal religion, and, later, against the new higher criticism of the Bible and Darwin's theory of natural selection. By the 19th century, fundamentalist thinking often included a commitment to premillennialism (the destruction of the world before Christ's second coming), and virtually everything, including mental illness, was understood in apocalyptic, premillennial terms: this sinful world would be destroyed in a horrific cataclysm, with only a saving remnant spared, and the devil and his forces would grow in power until the second coming when they would be destroyed by a triumphant Christ. There was no point then in trying to save insane persons, who were only a manifestation of the devil and thereby fulfilled the prophecies. Indeed, by the mid-19th century, to attempt to free "the insane" from the devil was contrary to premillennial views of a doomed American society. And for revivalists who were not premillennialist, the focus was on salvation, whatever the cost to mental stability: if one in a thousand of the newly saved went mad, it was a small price to pay.

Something of early, and influential, Calvinist religious stances toward insanity, especially in New England, can be seen in the attitudes of the most famous American philosopher-clergyman in the 18th century, and one of the most important philosophers in American history, Jonathan Edwards, and in those of his somewhat older contemporary and also a prominent Calvinist, the Reverend Cotton Mather. Mather, a prolific author who wrote also on medical and scientific subjects and was a member of the Royal Society, was yet a strong believer in witchcraft and the role of the devil in human affairs, and he considered sin to be the origin of insanity as of all illness, an old-fashioned view among physicians by the 1720s. Nevertheless, even *he* made exceptions. He noted that several clergymen had become insane not because of their sins but on the contrary because they served the Lord so well that the devil became enraged and drove them mad (Mather 1702/1967, pp. 438–442). Traditionally such a view would require admitting that the Lord, perhaps in order to test victims rather than punish them, had given the devil permission to work his will. Mather was apparently able to free from stigma at least some insane persons with whom he felt sympathy. He also considered his third wife mad, but whether from "a Distraction which may be somewhat Hereditary" or perhaps demonic possession, he could not say (Silverman 1985, p. 309). On the other hand he describes a critic of the clergy who after speaking in church was quickly and justifiably punished with madness (Wendell 1891, pp. 271–272).

Jonathan Edwards' view of insanity, while of long standing, did not arise from a deep interest in the subject or from much personal experience with the insane. During the first Great Awakening in 1735 Edwards preached sermons that intentionally terrified his audience. He dwelt on the dreadful fate in the pit of hell awaiting the unrepentant. Then tragedy did indeed strike. His uncle by marriage, Joseph Hawley, the leading merchant of Northampton, Massachusetts, committed suicide, an event that put a stop to religious excitement and conversations in the town and effectively ended the revival there. Edwards rationalized that his uncle had long been melancholic and greatly "concerned about the condition of his soul: till, by the ordering of a sovereign providence he was suffered to fall into a deep melancholy. . . . the devil took advantage and drove him into despairing thoughts," which led him to cut his throat (Edwards 1736/1972, p. 109). Why the "sovereign providence" saw fit to depress Hawley and give the devil an opportunity to suggest suicide was not explained. Edwards was at this time most concerned with the effect of this suicide upon the revival movement. He defended the revival and himself. "I have known," he wrote, "a very few instances of those, that in their great extremity (consequent to attending the revival meetings), have for a short space been deprived, in some measure of the use of reason; but among the many hundreds, and it may be thousands, that have lately been brought to such agonies, I never yet knew one, lastingly deprived of their [sic] reason." Religious enthusiasm is therefore not equivalent to insanity, nor does it cause that disorder. Besides, one must not temporize but tell the sinner the truth. "What of the thousands who commit suicides (from religious melancholy) after reading the Bible?" asks Edwards. Surely one would not therefore suggest suppressing God's word in order to prevent such suicides. At any rate thousands had been saved from eternal death by revivalist preaching. The view that the sinner was often a hardened reprobate who must be forced to seek salvation by sermons that terrified became the common outlook of revivalists. The highest good was salvation, and if some became insane in the process, that price was well worth the cost, for the result would be eternal life (Edwards 1736/1972, see pp. 224–265). This attitude persists in substance to the present among many religiously conservative, evangelical Protestants.

But like Mather, Edwards could free from stigma an afflicted person for whom he felt sympathy. In his later *Account of the Life of the Late Reverend Mr. David Brainerd*, recounting the life of a missionary to the Indians who was prone to melancholy, Edwards does not refer to Satan; instead Edwards attributes Brainerd's depression to natural causes. Edwards seems to have become aware that as long as melancholy, the term he used to include all degrees of mental upset from sadness to insanity, was seen as having a demonic component, many Christians would consider the afflicted as being punished for sins, a judgment he wished to avoid in the case of Brainerd (Parker 1968).

The persistent belief among some of the more religiously conservative evangelicals that people who were insane were irrational, violent, and immoral did not differ significantly from the general popular view (which of course had been influenced by religion). By the 19th century, this concept of insanity had diverged from that shared by several leading medical men who increasingly stressed that madness might exist without significant irrationality. Insanity, these physicians argued, might reveal itself more in moral disorder than irrationality, and behavior that the religious traditionally considered criminal, immoral, and sinful might actually be the consequence of insanity rather than components of it or indeed its cause. This issue remained for the 19th-century religious an area of disagreement with psychiatry, especially among many of the evangelical sects. As the former mental patient, Protestant minister, and psychologist Anton Boisen wrote in the 1930s, "The church has always taught that conviction of sin is the first step on the road to salvation" (Boisen 1952, p. 119). To the present, most of the Christian religious consider mankind fallen or at least "naturally" inclined to sin; recognition of sin has always been essential to accepting Christ, the acceptance of whom is the key to eternal life and ultimately more important than being cured of mental illness. If Christian conversion did not restore one to sanity or eliminate major emotional problems, at least the afflicted might more readily accept his or her fate and find solace and eternal life in Christ.

Nineteenth-century evangelical preachers remained committed to a literal interpretation of the Bible, which included demonic possession and miracle healing not only as a past event but as a present reality available to those who were true Christians. Sin remained the abiding explanation for the ills of mankind, including insanity. The attitude of Charles Grandison Finney, the most influential 19th-century revivalist, was typical.

Although he saw himself as fighting against Calvinism, Finney's views on insanity were virtually the same as Edwards'.[1] Thus, like Edwards, Finney expressed concern with insanity only incidentally as it threatened the revivalist movement. In 1835, during the second great revival movement, and almost exactly 100 years after Edwards wrote on the subject, Finney found himself accused of driving a woman communicant insane by insisting that she immediately accept his call and find Christ. Finney responded that the woman had become mad because she resisted his efforts to save her. Besides, the sinful were often intractable and had to be terrified into accepting salvation. Echoing Edwards' defense of revivalism after his uncle's suicide, Finney wrote:

---

[1]Finney, in fact, respected Edwards very much. Maintaining revivalistic fervor was all important to Finney: he thought that in the complacently Arminian days of the early 17th century, Edwards' determination Calvinism was the perfect formula, just as the complacent Calvinism of his own day demanded that he, Finney, preach free will in order to keep the revival going forward.

It is very common for persons to be waiting to be made subjects of prayer.
. . . They are so wicked, they say, that they can't come to Christ. They want to
try, by humiliation, and suffering, and prayer, to fit themselves to come. You
will have to hunt them out of all these refuges. It is astonishing into how many
corners they will often run before they will go to Christ. I have known persons
almost deranged for the want of a little correct instruction.

Finney's overweening faith in the power of the Word allowed him to see no
conflict between revivalism and psychiatry, but rather consanguinity: he
proclaimed that revivals saved many from madness and that untold numbers received eternal life, the most important gift of all. But as the power of
medicine and psychiatry grew, most evangelicals could no longer see themselves and psychiatrists and doctors as sharing common goals.

In contrast to the revivalists, the liberal Protestant clergy drastically
changed their image of insanity in the 19th century. Liberal Protestants
more and more agreed with the growing tendency of medicine and the at
that time new specialty of psychiatry to view insanity as a physical illness—
that is, a disorder whose symptoms and perhaps even sufficient causes were
mental but one that was essentially somatic, possibly a dysfunction of the
brain. A significant segment of the liberal clergy conceded to psychiatrists
the care of insane persons, with clergymen consigned to serve as chaplains
in the new mental hospitals being built under both private and state auspices all over the United States. As we have seen, the religious had always
been interested in insanity for its theological implications rather than out of
concern for the plight of the insane persons as such. What in effect seemed
to have happened was that many liberal clergymen, influenced in part by the
higher criticism of the Bible, abjuring fundamentalism and talk of the devil,
and eager to keep up with current scientific trends, came to ignore the
subject of insanity altogether as a religious theological issue. When in an
increasingly secular society psychiatrists won the predominant authority
over the treatment and management of mental illness, the liberal clergy
were ready to accept them as the experts on the subject.

Indeed, late 19th- and early 20th-century Christians who did not insist
upon a literal and inerrant interpretation of the Bible consistently tried to
reconcile their religious beliefs with psychiatry. Some simply accepted a
naturalistic explanation of insanity, while others sought to retain a role for
the supernatural. One trend was to revive the cure of souls or establish the
practice of pastoral counseling. The burden of this trend, which began with
the Emmanuel Movement in Boston in the early 20th century, was to bring
people to health by using psychotherapy in a process of reconciling patients
with Christ while at the same time attempting to alleviate their symptoms.
But even within the Emmanuel Movement a patient who was the equivalent of what later would be called the "psychotic" patient would be sent to
psychiatrists for treatment, so that in theory no significant challenge was

posed to psychiatry, albeit the cure of souls or pastoral therapy constituted in effect competition with psychiatry. And despite Freud's open atheism, some liberal Protestants and even Catholics accepted psychoanalysis—properly modified to include sin (often in place of Freud's concept of guilt)—as the preferred means of dealing with the emotional upsets of church members. Many liberal Protestants thought psychoanalysis provided the most penetrating examination of human nature yet conceived; even more, they believed that the knowledge derived from Freud's work was essential to understanding human motivation and therefore also essential to advancing the cause of Christianity in the modern world.

As in the case of Cotton Mather, even those firmly convinced that sin caused insanity thought there were exceptions. There were implicit class and social attitudes at work, as well as familial ties, in the distinctions Mather made between the sinful and blameworthy and the innocent. Boisen's writing in the 20th century is not too different. He makes clear that he seeks to help the "worthy" insane, those struggling to resolve problems of life and death and of instinctual drives (mainly sexual). These are the kind of people whom religion can help; by implication, they would tend to be educated and therefore middle or upper class (Boisen 1952). The idea that certain patients either deserved or could benefit better from treatment, religious or psychiatric, than other patients was of course not confined to the religious but was widespread in the psychiatric profession and society at large from the time when mental hospitals were first built in British North America in the late 18th century. Indeed, despite the fact that in law and by common consent among at least the educated public, insane persons were not held responsible for their actions, the view of all concerned was in fact significantly influenced not only by the class and social status of the insane person but also by his or her symptomatology and previous moral character. The pious individual who became insane might be freed from blame and minimally stigmatized by his or her disorder; the reprobate was likely not to be thus spared. And if the now insane person committed no outrageous acts, and his or her religious beliefs and moral standards remained intact, the chances for absolution from sin would be good.

But this is far from the whole story. In the late 19th century new Christian sects appeared, most notably Christian Science and Jehovah's Witnesses—all of which tended to blame the victim. Christian Science argues that disease is a consequence of wrong belief; the afflicted are responsible, by way of their inadequate faith, for their misfortune and their inability to recover. Jehovah's Witnesses, stressing the belief that sin and the devil cause insanity, tend to reject mentally troubled members. The formation of an organized fundamentalist movement in the 1920s and the prominence in our own time of Pentecostals and charismatics have perpetuated the view of insane persons as sinful and responsible for their disorder. The biblical view, as interpreted by these groups, stresses the role of sin as the cause of insanity, with the devil playing his traditional role and exorcism and miracles remaining the chief means by which to restore those possessed by evil spirits. In this view the possessed are irrational, violent, immoral, sinful, and faithless people being punished for their sins or for their lack of faith. Exorcism and repentance are the only way out.

The irony is that Christian Scientists, Jehovah's Witnesses, fundamentalists, Pentecostals, and charismatics were (and are) not much concerned with the insane or psychotic individual, whom they, like their liberal religionist opponents, have sent to psychiatrists for treatment. Until very recently insanity was seldom discussed in most Protestant religious literature. And even the recent growth of religious interest in the emotional problems of communicants has not generally extended to those mentally troubled enough to be unable to care for themselves, the so-called psychotics, who are left to psychiatry by liberal Protestants who believe that they do not have the expertise to treat them. Conservative, fundamentalist Protestants frequently condemn psychiatry, but because they make almost no provision for the disturbed parishioners who do not recover despite exorcism, the latter persons end up in public institutions or on the streets, duly punished for their sins or their lack of faith, and hence by default consigned to the secular domain.

The persistence of stigmatizing mentally disturbed people as sinful and personally blameworthy for their disorder cannot be accounted for simply as a long-held Christian belief. It is perhaps more important that to many Protestant clergy a challenge to the biblical concept of insanity seems to be a challenge to Christianity itself. Conservative Christians seem to believe that to abandon the idea that sin and the devil are the origin of most psychoses would be to deny the clearly stated views of Christ as reported in the New Testament and thus to deny the Bible as an inerrant source of all valid Christian belief. Even liberal Protestant clergy find this subject problematical. If mankind is not innately sinful, how can the role of organized religion as moral arbiter be justified and what of the traditional view of the role of Christ in freeing mankind of sin? The implication is that the insane are more guilty of sin than others, and if so, in some sense insanity is punishment for sin. But clergymen commenting on their role in the cure of souls not uncommonly remark that they cannot compete with psychiatrists as specialists in therapy. Thus by in practice abandoning the seriously ill to psychiatry, the religious maintain their historical emphasis on conversion, with its potential to bolster faith and/or the literal accuracy of the Bible, rather than therapy. In a sense, then, Christianity, liberal or conservative, symbolic or literal, has a basic problem with associating mental illness with sin, a problem that in practical terms has been resolved by rendering the afflicted unto Caesar.

References

Boisen AT: The Exploration of the Inner World: A Study of Mental Disorder and Religious Experience. New York, Harper Torchbooks, 1952

Edwards J: The Great Awakening: A Faithful Narrative . . . (1736). Edited by Goen CC. New Haven, CT, Yale University Press, 1972

Finney CG: Lectures on Revivals of Religion . . . , 2nd Edition. New York, AS Barnes, 1835

Mather C: Magnolia Christi Americana: The Ecclesiastical History of New England (1702). New York, Russell & Russell, 1967

Neaman JS: Suggestion of the Devil: The Origin of Madness. Garden City, NY, Anchor Books/Doubleday, 1975

Parker GT: Jonathan Edwards and melancholy. New England Quarterly 41(June):193–212, 1968

Silverman K: The Life and Times of Cotton Mather. New York, Columbia University Press, 1985

Wendell B: Cotton Mather, the Puritan Priest. New York, Dodd, Mead, 1891

Further Reading

Beall OT Jr, Shryock R: Cotton Mather: First Significant Figure in American Medicine. Baltimore, MD, Johns Hopkins University Press, 1954

The Beginnings of Mental Hygiene in America: Three Selected Essays, 1833–1850. New York, Arno Press, 1973

Bergsten G: Pastoral Psychology: A Study in the Care of Souls. London, Allen and Unwin, 1951

Biddle WE: Integration of Religion and Psychiatry. New York, Collier Books, 1962

Bonomi PU: Under the Cope of Heaven: Religion, Society, and Politics in Colonial America. New York, Oxford University Press, 1986

Boorse C: On the distinction between disease and illness. Philosophy & Public Affairs 5:49–68, 1975

Boorse C: Health as a theoretical concept. Philosophy of Science 44:542–573, 1977

Bowker J: Problems of Suffering in the Religions of the World. Cambridge, UK, Cambridge University Press, 1970

Bozeman TD: Protestants in an Age of Science: The Baconian Ideal and Antebellum American Religious Thought. Chapel Hill, NC, University of North Carolina Press, 1977

Braceland FJ (ed): Faith, Reason and Modern Psychiatry: Sources for a Synthesis. New York, PJ Kenedy, 1955

Braden CS: Christian Science Today: Power, Policy, Practice. Dallas, TX, Southern Methodist University Press, 1958

Braden CS: Spirits in Rebellion: The Rise and Development of New Thought. Dallas, TX, Southern Methodist University Press, 1963

Brigham A: Observations on the Influence of Religion Upon the Health and Physical Welfare of Mankind (1835). New York, Arno Press, 1973

Brigham A: Remarks on the Influence of Mental Cultivation and Mental Excitement Upon Health, 2nd Edition. Boston, MA, Marsh, Capen & Lyon, 1833

Brown R: Demonology and Witchcraft. . . . London, John F Shaw, 1889

Caporale R, Grumelli A (eds): The Culture of Unbelief: Studies and Proceedings From the First International Symposium on Belief. Berkeley, CA, University of California Press, 1971

A Century of Christian Science Healing. Boston, MA, Christian Science Publishing Society, 1966

Clebsch WA, Jaekle CR: Pastoral Care in Historical Perspective. New York, Jason Aronson, 1964

Dain N: Concepts of Insanity in the United States, 1789–1865. New Brunswick, NJ, Rutgers University Press, 1964

Dillenberger J: Protestant Thought and Natural Science: A Historical Interpretation. Garden City, NY, Doubleday, 1960

Eddy MB: The First Church of Christ Scientist and Miscellany. Boston, MA, The Trustees under the Will of Mary Baker G Eddy, 1941

Edwards J: The Life of David Brainerd. Edited by Norman Pettit. New Haven, CT, Yale University Press, 1985

Feilding A: Faith-Healing and "Christian Science." London, Duckworth, 1899

Finney CG: Memoirs. New York, AS Barnes, 1876

Flake C: Redemptorama: Culture, Politics, and the New Evangelicalism. Garden City, NY, Anchor Books/Doubleday, 1984

Foskett J: Meaning in Madness: The Pastor and the Mentally Ill. New Library of Pastoral Care. London, SPCK, 1984

Fuller RC: Mesmerism and the American Cure of Souls. Philadelphia, PA, University of Pennsylvania Press, 1982

Fuller RC: Americans and the Unconscious. New York, Oxford University Press, 1986

Fuller RC: Alternative Medicine and American Religious Life. New York, Oxford University Press, 1989

Goldbrunner J: Cure of Mind and Cure of Soul: Depth Psychology and Pastoral Care. Translated from the German 2nd Edition by Godman S. Notre Dame, IN, University of Notre Dame Press, 1962

Gross L: God and Freud. New York, David McKay, 1959

Harrison BG: Visions of Glory: A History and a Memory of Jehovah's Witnesses. New York, Simon and Schuster, 1978

Heimert A: Religion and the American Mind: From the Great Awakening to the Revolution. Cambridge, MA, Harvard University Press, 1966

Hepworth M, Turner BS: Confession: Studies in Deviance and Religion. London, Routledge & Kegan Paul, 1982

Hovenkamp H: Science and Religion in America, 1800–1860. Philadelphia, PA, University of Pennsylvania Press, 1978

Hulme WE: Theology and counseling. Christian Century 60(Feb 21):238–239, 1951

Hunter JD: Evangelicalism: The Coming Generation. Chicago, IL, University of Chicago Press, 1987

Kelsey MT: Healing and Christianity in Ancient Thought and Modern Times. New York, Harper & Row, 1973

Kelsey MT: Tongue Speaking: An Experiment in Spiritual Experience. Garden City, NY, Doubleday, 1964

Knox RA: Enthusiasm: A Chapter in the History of Religion, With Special Reference to the XVII and XVIII centuries. Oxford, UK, Clarendon Press, 1959

Leuba JH: The Psychology of Religious Mysticism. New York, Harcourt, Brace, 1929

Linberg DC, Number RL: God and Nature: Historical Essays on the Encounter Between Christianity and Science. Berkeley, CA, University of California Press, 1986

Maloney HN, Lovekin AA: Glossolalia: Behavioral Science Perspectives on Speaking in Tongues. New York, Oxford University Press, 1985

Marsden GM: Fundamentalism and American Culture: The Shaping of Twentieth-Century Evangelicalism, 1870-1925. Oxford, UK, Oxford University Press, 1980

Marsden GM (ed): Evangelicalism and Modern America. Grand Rapids, MI, William B Eerdman, 1984

Martin M: Hostage to the Devil: The Possession and Exorcism of Five Living Americans. New York, Harper & Row, 1987

Marvin AP: The Life and Times of Cotton Mather, D.D., F.R.S.; or, A Boston Minister of Two Centuries Ago, 1663-1728. Boston, MA, Congregational Sunday-School and Publishing Society, 1892

Mather C: The Wonders of the Invisible World; Being an Account of the Tryals of Several Witches Lately Executed in New-England. London, John Russell Smith, 1862

Mather C: Bonifacius: An Essay Upon the Good. Edited by Levin D. Cambridge, MA, Belknap Press/Harvard University Press, 1966

Mather C: The Angel of Bethesda. Edited by Jones GW. Barre, MA, American Antiquarian Society and Barre Publishers, 1972

McLoughlin WG Jr: Modern Revivalism: Charles Grandison Finney to Billy Graham. New York, Ronald Press, 1959

McNeill JT: A History of the Cure of Souls. New York, Harper & Row, 1951

Meissner WW: Psychoanalysis and Religious Experience. New Haven, CT, Yale University Press, 1984

Meyer D: The Positive Thinkers: Religion as Pop Psychology From Mary Baker Eddy to Oral Roberts. New York, Pantheon, 1980

Moore RL: In Search of White Crows: Spiritualism, Parapsychology and American Culture. New York, Oxford University Press, 1977

Moore RL: Religious Outsiders and the Making of Americans. New York, Oxford University Press, 1986

Mowrer OH: The Crisis in Psychiatry and Religion. Princeton, NJ, Van Nostrand Co, 1961

Mowrer OH (ed): Morality and Mental Health. Chicago, IL, Rand McNally, 1967

Murray JAC: An Introduction to a Christian Psycho-therapy. New York, Scribner's, 1938

Neussberm WW: Psychoanalysis and Religious Experience. New Haven, CT, Yale University Press, 1984

Palmer PF: Sacraments and Forgiveness: History and Doctrinal Development of Penance, Extreme Unction and Indulgences. Sources of Christian Theology, Vol 2. London, 1959

Pattison EM, Lapins N, Doerr HA: Faith healing: a study of personality and function. J Nerv Ment Dis 157:397-409, 1973

Penton MJ: Apocalypse Delayed: The Story of Jehovah's Witnesses. Toronto, University of Toronto Press, 1985

Poloma M: The Charismatic Movement: Is There a New Pentecost? Boston, MA, Twayne, 1982

Russell JB: The Devil and Perceptions of Evil From Antiquity to Primitive Christianity. Ithaca, NY, Cornell University Press, 1977

Scull A: Social Order/Mental Disorder: Anglo-American Psychiatry in Historical Perspective. Berkeley, CA, University of California Press, 1989

Stokes GA: Ministry after Freud: the rise of the religion and health movement in American protestantism, 1906–1945. Unpublished doctoral dissertation, Yale University, New Haven, CT, 1981

Stolz NR: The Church and Psychotherapy. New York, Abingdon-Cokesbury Press, 1943

Tentler TN: Sin and Confession on the Eve of the Reformation. Princeton, NJ, Princeton University Press, 1977

Thomas K: Religion and the Decline of Magic. New York, Scribner's, 1970

Turner BS: Confession: Studies in Deviance and Religion. Boston, MA, Routledge & Kegan Paul, 1982

Turner J: Without God, Without Creed: The Origins of Unbelief in America. Baltimore, MD, Johns Hopkins University Press, 1985

Upham CW: Salem Witchcraft and Cotton Mather: A Reply. Morrisania, NY, 1869

Walker DP: Unclean Spirits: Possession and Exorcism in France and England in the Late Sixteenth and Early Seventeenth Centuries. Philadelphia, PA, University of Pennsylvania Press, 1981

Weatherhead LD: Psychology, Religion and Healing. London, Hodder and Stoughton, 1951

Weisman R: Witchcraft, Magic, and Religion in 17th-Century Massachusetts. Amherst, MA, University of Massachusetts Press, 1984

Worcester E, McComb S, Coriat IH: Religion and Medicine: The Moral Control of Nervous Disorders. New York, Moffat, Yard, 1908

Zaretsky II, Leone MP (eds): Religious Movements in Contemporary America. Princeton, NJ, Princeton University Press, 1974

Societal Issues

The Consequences of Stigma for Persons With Mental Illness: Evidence From the Social Sciences

Bruce G. Link, Ph.D.
Francis T. Cullen, Ph.D.
Jerold Mirotznik, Ph.D.
Elmer Struening, Ph.D.

During the past two decades sociologists and social psychologists have become increasingly interested in stigma itself as an area of study (Archer 1985). They have studied the stigma of many conditions and compared and contrasted the dimensions of stigma across these different conditions (Jones et al. 1984). These researchers are interested in stigma not simply because of its effects on the stigmatized but because of what it reveals about social interaction and about the society we live in. Theoretical perspectives are constructed about the nature of stigma, about what causes it, and about the consequences it can have (Goffman 1963; Jones et al. 1984; Link et al. 1989). The potential value of this broad theoretical approach for studying the stigma associated with any single type of stigmatized condition is that it offers the opportunity to deepen our understanding of how stigma works for that condition. In this chapter we review the social science literature as it bears on the stigma of mental illness. As we will see, this literature embodies sharply divergent views about the importance of stigma in mental illness.

Stigma Defined

Erving Goffman (1963, p. 3) characterized "stigma" as an attribute that is socially defined as "deeply discrediting." More recently, Jones et al. (1984)

defined stigma in a two-part sequence. First, there must be what Jones et al. call a "mark" or a "deviation from a prototype or a norm" that might be stigmatizing (p. 8). Then, echoing Goffman, the authors indicate that to be stigmatizing a mark must link the bearer to unwanted, usually undesirable attributes that discredit him or her in the eyes of others. For example, if a person is hospitalized for mental illness and is then assumed to be dangerous, incompetent, or untrustworthy, the person, according to this definition, is stigmatized. This definition highlights the main issue characterizing the debate over stigma in the social science literature. Are people who have sought help for mental illness stigmatized as a consequence? Does being marked a "mental patient" or a "psychiatric patient" induce stigma?

The Importance of Stigma for Mentally Ill Persons: Contrasting Views

The debate over the importance of stigma in mental illness could hardly be more sharply drawn. One side in the debate argues that research refutes the proposition that mentally ill persons are stigmatized. Sociologist Walter Gove (1982), for example, claims that "[m]ost mental patients experience some stigma; however, in the vast majority of cases the stigma appears to be transitory and does not appear to pose a significant problem" (p. 280). Crocetti et al. (1974) contend that former patients "enjoy nearly total acceptance in all but the most intimate relationships" (p. 88). For these authors, the continuing belief in the stigma of mental illness is so blind to the facts and so misguided that it must be explained in other ways. "Many psychiatrists," Crocetti et al. contend, "from time to time, experience hostility from the rest of the medical community toward their specialty. Some psychiatrists are quite sensitive to real and imagined prejudice by their medical colleagues. With these therapists, the danger of identifying with the patient as a victim of an equally rejecting community is ever present" (p. 134). However, other research sharply challenges these conclusions by showing how the data on which these conclusions were based were either methodologically biased or else too narrow in scope to assess the powerful force that stigma can be in the lives of people who suffer from mental illness. Below we first present the evidence that has led some to deny the importance of stigma. We then follow this by discussing the more recent research that has reaffirmed the importance of stigma.

Why Some Social Scientists Believe Stigma Is Unimportant

Three general types of evidence have been used to support the conclusion that stigma is unimportant in the lives of mentally ill persons. The first comes from survey research on public attitudes toward persons with mental illness. In this research members of the public are asked whether they would be willing to interact with a former mental patient in a variety of relationships. For example, respondents are asked, "How would you feel about working on the same job with someone who has been mentally ill?" and "Can you imagine falling in love with someone who has been mentally ill?" Those who believe the impact of stigma is unimportant argue that public attitudes, as represented by accepting responses to questions like these, are too positive to sustain the notion that former mental patients face rejection from community members. In fact when Crocetti et al. (1974) asked a sample of automobile factory workers a similar set of questions, they found that most individuals were willing to work on the same job (94%), room with (64%), or even fall in love with (54%) a person who had been mentally ill. Based on these results and ones like them Crocetti et al. concluded that "[a]s defined by social-distance scales the mentally ill simply are not subject to prejudice even vaguely related to racial prejudice. In fact, neither our study [n]or other recent studies document the presence of clear prejudice toward those who have been mentally ill" (pp. 88–89).

A second source of data that has led some social scientists to conclude that stigma is an unimportant factor comes from experimental studies that vary "labeling" and "behavior." In these studies members of the public are asked to react to "vignettes" (either written or acted) in which conditions of "labeling" (former mental patient vs. no mention of mental illness) and behavior (normal vs. indicative of mental illness) are experimentally manipulated. In 12 of the 15 studies of this type that we were able to locate, aberrant behavior was a stronger determinant of rejection than was the label of "former mental patient" (Link et al. 1987). Moreover, the effect of knowing that someone had been a mental patient had little effect on responses in many studies.

These studies have had a powerful influence on thinking about stigma. For example, Rabkin, a frequent reviewer of the literature on attitudes toward mental illness, has reported that a 1980 National Institute of Mental Health workshop of experts in the field decided not to use the term "stigma" in the title of its proceedings. Apparently, stigma was not viewed as an appropriate designation if "one is referring to negative attitudes induced by manifestations of psychiatric illness" (p. 327). The conclusion as represented in the workshop proceedings seems to be that if people who have been mental patients behave in a bizarre fashion they will be rejected, but if they behave normally they face little stigma.

The third source of data that has led some researchers to dismiss the importance of stigma is surveys of mental patients. These surveys indicate that patients and former patients are rarely able to report concrete instances of rejection (Gove and Fain 1973; Huffine and Clausen 1979). Moreover, many studies have asked patients about their attitudes toward their experiences in mental hospitals and in the community after leaving the hospital. Based on a review of 35 such studies, Weinstein (1983) concluded that patients do not feel uniformly stigmatized and tend to view their treatment by mental health professionals favorably.

In summary, these sources imply that public attitudes are accepting, and if rejection of former patients does occur, it is much more likely to be due to disturbed behavior than to stigma. When patient attitudes are assessed, many report being relatively unaffected by stigma.

Evidence Documenting the Importance of Stigma

Despite the seemingly persuasive case that can be made challenging the importance of stigma, each of the pieces of information that has been used to bolster this view can be shown to be lacking. This information is lacking because it either inappropriately underestimates the importance of stigma because of methodological problems or it fails to investigate the more subtle ways in which stigma affects those with mental illness.

Are attitudes benign? Consider first the research that is based on asking the public in a straightforward manner their attitudes about interacting with a former mental patient (Crocetti et al. 1974). The problem, of course, is the hypothetical nature of the questions—there is no flesh-and-blood mental patient asking, for example, to rent a room in one's home—which allows the respondent to give a socially desirable answer and compromises our ability to take answers to questions like these at face value. Evidence that this in fact occurs derives from an experiment conducted by Link and Cullen (1983). They questioned the notion that respondent reports can be regarded as true indicators of the rejection patients encounter. Link and Cullen did this by randomly assigning to community respondents different ways of asking social-distance questions about a person described in a vignette. Some were asked whether they thought an "ideal person" would allow contact with a former patient, whereas others were asked whether they themselves would allow such contact, and still others were asked whether most people would. The results showed that when a vignette was "labeled" by including a reference to a history of mental hospitalization, the "ideal person" way of asking questions produced the most acceptance, followed by the "self" mode, with the "most people" way of asking questions producing the most rejecting responses. Apparently, community residents know that the socially desirable response to a former patient is one of acceptance (i.e., an ideal person would be accepting). When subjects were asked whether they would accept the former patient, responses fell between this ideal and their perception of how most people respond. For respondents randomly assigned to unlabeled vignettes, the results were quite different. In this instance there was no reference to mental hospitalization to suggest the salience of the idea that one should be accepting of the described person. The results show that subjects who answered social-distance questions about their own attitudes were more rejecting than those answering either the "ideal" or "most people" questions. Together, this evidence suggests that people respond in a socially desirable way when reporting their own attitudes about a group they have learned they "should" accept. It calls into question conclusions about the benign nature of public attitudes based on the frequency of "accepting" responses to straightforward social-distance items.

Another challenge to the claim that attitudes are benign comes from studies that compare mental illness to other potentially stigmatizing conditions. Albrecht et al. (1982) have shown that "mental illness" is one of the most highly rejected conditions, clustering with drug addiction, prostitution, and ex-convict status rather than with cancer, diabetes, and heart disease (also see Tringo 1970). In another study, Lamy (1966) asked respondents to compare former mental hospital patients to exconvicts. He found that 1) respondents viewed the former mental patient role as even less desirable than the exconvict role, 2) respondents thought mothers would be more likely to trust an exconvict with the care of their children than a former mental patient, and 3) an exconvict would be much more reliable in an emergency than would a former mental patient. When a comparative approach is employed, public attitudes do not appear to be nearly as favorable as was claimed by Crocetti et al. (1974), whose data were almost certainly skewed by respondents giving socially desirable answers.

Finally, a few studies have investigated how people respond in situations where they are personally involved—circumstances that are much less likely to induce socially desirable responses. For example, Page (1977) obtained a sample of advertisements for apartments to rent and randomly assigned landlords to different conditions. In some conditions a caller working with Page's research team indicated that he was a patient in a mental hospital who would be released in a day or two, whereas in a control condition no mention of mental hospitalization was made. When mental patient status was known, landlords were much less likely to indicate that the apartment was available (27%) than in the control condition (83%).

Is it deviant behavior or stigma that causes rejection? Consider next the claim that it is the deviant behavior associated with mental illness, not the stigma itself, that leads to rejection. Work on the "self-fulfilling prophecy" in social psychology shows the dramatic effect that even a relatively benign mental illness label can exert in the absence of any deviant behavior whatsoever. Sibicky and Dovidio (1986) randomly assigned 68 male and 68 female introductory psychology students as mixed sex pairs to one of two conditions. In one condition, a "perceiver" (randomly assigned) was led to believe that a "target" was recruited from the psychological therapy clinic at the college. In the other condition, the perceiver was led to believe the individual was a fellow student in introductory psychology. In fact the target was always recruited from the class, and both targets and perceivers were led to believe that the study involved "the acquaintance process in social interaction." Each member of a pair completed a brief inventory of their courses, hobbies, and activities. Then the experimenter exchanged the inventories and provided the perceiver with the labeling information (student or therapy client). Subsequently, the two engaged in a tape-recorded interaction that was later reliably evaluated by two raters blind to the experimental conditions. Even before meeting them, perceivers rated the therapy targets less favorably. Moreover, the judges' ratings revealed that in their interactions with therapy targets, perceivers were less open, secure, sensitive, and sincere. Finally, the results showed that the behavior of the therapy targets was adversely affected as well, even though the targets had no knowledge of the experimental manipulation. Thus, expectations associated with being in psychological therapy color subsequent interactions, actually evoking certain behavior that confirms those expectations.

Another study has raised doubts about the notion that only deviant behavior, and not stigma, produces rejection. Link et al. (1987) began by reviewing the experimental or quasi-experimental studies comparing the relative importance of a mental illness label and deviant behavior. Recall that most of these studies showed that behavior is more important than a mental illness label in eliciting negative social reactions, a fact that led many to conclude that stigma was unimportant. Link et al. noted, however, that none of these studies made an attempt to assess what the label "former mental patient" meant to the respondents in the studies.

As a result, the authors conducted a study that sought to incorporate a measure of the extent to which people believed that mental patients in general were "dangerous." By conducting a vignette experiment similar to the ones they reviewed, they tested the idea that labeling could make these beliefs relevant to a person's acceptance. The experiment varied labeling (past mental hospitalization versus hospitalization for a back problem) and deviant behavior. A social-distance scale was used as an outcome measure.

The data analysis indicated that when the vignette described a subject without a mental illness label, beliefs about the dangerousness of mentally ill persons played no part in determining social-distancing responses to the person described in the vignette. When the vignette described a labeled subject, however, these beliefs became a potent determinant of responses. This pattern of results held regardless of the degree of deviant behavior. In fact, Link et al. were able to show that beliefs about dangerousness that were activated by labeling were just as strong predictors of social-distance responses as were variations in behavior. Apparently a mental illness label activates beliefs about the dangerousness of mental patients, making such beliefs important for determining how much social distance a person desires from a "former mental patient." Finally, it should be noted that if Link et al. had proceeded without bringing the measure of perceived dangerousness into the analysis—and thus achieved a more complete specification of stigma processes—they too would have found large effects of behavior and no effects of stigma.

Another challenge to the idea that only behavior—and not stigma—is important in producing rejection is provided by two ingenious studies conducted by Farina and his colleagues (1968, 1971). These studies show that stigma can produce the kind of behavior that others find objectionable. In experiments with patients and nonpatients, Farina and his colleagues randomly assigned subjects to one of two conditions. In one, subjects believed that a person with whom they were about to interact had been told that the subjects had at one time been hospitalized. In the other, the subjects believed that this person had no such knowledge. Even though the partners in interaction were always given the same neutral information, the subjects who believed that the other person knew about their hospitalization behaved in ways that evoked negative responses.

Are patients unconcerned about stigma?   While studies involving patient attitudes have been used to suggest that a mental illness label is not particularly stigmatizing, there are good reasons to question this conclusion.

Most important, the studies are hardly uniform in indicating that patients are unconcerned with matters of stigma. In his review of 35 studies on patient attitudes Weinstein (1983) found five dealing explicitly with patients views of stigma, three of which he classified as "unfavorable"—that is, as indicating that stigma is perceived as a problem by patients. Moreover, even within the two studies deemed favorable there were significant indications that some patients, though not a majority, felt intensely stigmatized. For example, in one of the two "favorable" studies the authors provided the following verbatim quote from a patient: "I don't think it makes any difference how often you come in. I think once you've been there (in the hospital) and they know you've been there, they call you crazy or sick" (Rosenblatt and Mayer 1974). Thus, while it is true that patients do not uniformly feel stigmatized, it is also true that many do feel this way, sometimes intensely so.

Moreover, while clearly relevant to stigma, the studies reviewed by Weinstein failed to tap some of the theoretically most important attitudes that patients might hold. In particular, patients were not asked their perceptions of how other people perceive mental patients, or whether other people would stigmatize them. Link and his colleagues (1989) investigated this in a sample of respondents from outpatient clinics and inpatient facilities in the Washington Heights section of New York City. When asked whether they thought most people would exclude a mental patient from a close friendship, a job, or an intimate relationship, a large majority of respondents indicated that they believed this would indeed happen. Thus, there is a generalized expectation among patients that most people will devalue and discriminate against them, a belief that has potent consequences.

How Stigma Affects Mentally Ill Persons

Despite the studies mentioned in the foregoing step-by-step response to those who believe stigma is unimportant, a gap in the literature has remained. If stigma is important, then those who believe it to be so should be able to specify how stigma affects "real world" aspects of mental patients' lives. In this regard Link (1987) has offered an explanation that identifies a mechanism by which patient attitudes about stigma may strongly affect their life circumstances. He argues that a mental illness label gives personal relevance to an individual's beliefs about how *most* people respond to mental patients. According to this view, people develop conceptions of what others think of mental patients long *before* they themselves ever become patients. These conceptions are often quite negative both among the general public and, as we have just reported, among mental patients (Link 1987; Link et al. 1989). Link notes that such beliefs take on new relevance when nonpatients become psychiatric patients for the first time. What once seemed to be an innocuous array of beliefs about people's attitudes toward mental patients is now applicable personally and takes on new meaning. Being marked a mental patient transforms a person's beliefs about the devaluation and discrimination of mental patients into a personal expectation of rejection. Once patients expect rejection, the theory goes, interactions with others may be strained and strategies aimed at minimizing the rejection they fear—such as withdrawing from social contacts—may impair their ability to function. In this approach it is not the direct negative reactions of others that produce harmful consequences but rather the internalization of the expected reactions. Thus, negative labeling effects can arise because of processes that operate through the attitudes and behaviors of patients.

To test this explanation Link (1987) constructed a 12-item scale measuring the extent to which a person believes that mental patients will be devalued and discriminated against. This scale was administered to both mental patients and nonmental patients in an epidemiological "case control" study of major depression and schizophrenia. Link showed that the degree to which a person expects to be rejected is associated with demoralization, income loss, and unemployment in individuals labeled mentally ill but not in individuals not labeled as such, thereby supporting the notion that labeling activates beliefs that lead to negative consequences.

In recent work Link et al. (1989) extend the foregoing reasoning in two ways. First, they bring into the analysis, empirical measures of the coping strategies of secrecy (concealing a history of treatment), withdrawal (avoiding potentially threatening situations), and education (attempting to teach others in order to forestall the negative effects of stereotypes). Consistent with the notion that the stigma of mental illness labeling activates expectations of rejection, the authors show that patients tend to endorse these strategies as a means of protecting themselves. Second, they extend the analysis to a consideration of the effects of stigmatization on social network ties. Patients who fear rejection most and who endorse the strategy of withdrawal have insular support networks consisting mainly of household members.

Conclusion

Taken together, the evidence suggests strongly that there *are* negative consequences that follow from stigma. The studies that lead us to this conclusion have varied in design and have been conducted in a variety of samples, using many different types of outcome measures. Moreover, these studies show why the evidence used to discount the effects of stigma is biased by socially desirable responses or is too limited in complexity to adequately test stigma and its consequences. We conclude that stigma has significant effects on many important aspects of patients lives. We believe that future research on stigma should set aside the question of whether stigma is important. This question has dominated too much research for too long. Instead, we need to ask, "How can we overcome stigma?"

References

Albrecht G, Walker V, Levy J: Social distance from the stigmatized: a test of two theories. Soc Sci Med 16:1319–1327, 1982

Archer D: Social deviance, in The Handbook of Social Psychology, Vol 2. Edited by Lindsay G. Aronson E. New York, Random House, 1985, pp 743–804

Crocetti G, Spiro H, Siassi I: Contemporary Attitudes Towards Mental Illness. Pittsburgh, PA, University of Pittsburgh Press, 1974

Farina A, Allen J, Saul B: The role of the stigmatized person in effecting social relationships. J Pers 36:169–182, 1968

Farina A, Gliha D, Boudreau L, et al: Mental illness and the impact of believing others know about it. J Abnorm Psychol 77:1–5, 1971

Goffman I: Stigma: Notes on the Management of Spoiled Identity. Englewood Cliffs, NJ, Prentice-Hall, 1963

Gove WR: The current status of the labeling theory of mental illness, in Deviance and Mental Illness. Edited by Gove WR. Beverly Hills, CA, Sage, 1982, pp 273–300

Gove W, Fain T: The stigma of mental hospitalization: an attempt to evaluate its consequences. Arch Gen Psychiatry 29:494–500, 1973

Huffine C, Clausen J: Madness and work: short- and long-term effects of mental illness on occupational careers. Social Forces 57:1049–1062, 1979

Jones E, Farina A, Markus H, et al: Social Stigma: The Psychology of Marked Relationships. New York, WH Freeman, 1984

Lamy RE: Social consequences of mental illness. J Consult Clin Psychol 30:450–455, 1966

Link BG: Understanding labeling effects in the area of mental disorders: an assessment of the effects of expectations of rejection. American Sociological Review 52:96–112, 1987

Link BG, Cullen FT: Reconsidering the social rejection of ex-mental patients: levels of attitudinal response. Am J Community Psychol 11:261–273, 1983

Link BG, Cullen FT, Frank J, et al: The social rejection of former mental patients: understanding why labels matter. American Journal of Sociology 92:1461–1500, 1987

Link BG, Cullen FT, Struening EL, et al: A modified labeling theory approach to mental disorders and empirical assessment. American Sociological Review 54:400–423, 1989

Page S: Effects of the mental illness label in attempts to obtain accommodation. Canadian Journal of Behavioral Sciences 9:85–90, 1977

Rabkin J: Determinants of public attitudes about mental illness: summary of research literature, in Attitudes Toward the Mentally Ill: Research Perspectives (DHHS Publ No ADM-80-1031). Edited by Rabkin J, Gelb L, Lazar J. Bethesda, MD, National Institute of Mental Health

Rosenblatt A, Mayer J: Patients who return: a consideration of some neglected influences. Journal of the Bronx State Hospital 2:71–81, 1974

Sibicky M, Dovidio J: Stigma of psychological therapy: stereotypes, interpersonal reactions, and the self-fulfilling prophecy. J Consult Clin Psychol 33:148–154, 1986

Tringo J: The hierarchy of preference toward disability groups. Journal of Special Education 4:295–306, 1970

Weinstein R: Labeling theory and the attitudes of mental patients: a review. J Health Soc Behav 24:70–84, 1983

Chapter 10

Stigma and Stereotype: Homeless Mentally Ill Persons

William R. Breakey, M.D.
Pamela J. Fischer, Ph.D.
Gerald Nestadt, M.D.
Alan Romanoski, M.D.

Homeless mentally ill persons are doubly stigmatized. As homeless people, they are perceived as failures in a success-oriented society. In addition, they are portrayed as the bizarre products of deinstitutionalization, discharged from the hospitals onto the streets.

The Baltimore Homeless Study revealed that many stereotypes of homeless individuals are not true. People who are homeless are not primarily transients; they are not dirty and lice-infested. They are people in poor health, on the fringe of society.

Because stigma is fostered by ignorance, the development and dissemination of knowledge about mental illness and homelessness is one vital effort in the campaign to reduce stigma.

On a stormy night in Baltimore, a homeless mentally ill man, a patient of Baltimore's Health Care for the Homeless program, took shelter in an abandoned building scheduled for demolition and reconstruction as a women's shelter. The storm was severe enough that parts of the building collapsed, killing the man. Newspaper reports of this tragedy described the victim as a "drifter." Other words could have been used: "bum," "wino," "vagrant," "tramp," or in the case of a woman, "bag lady." Any of these terms would serve the function of stereotyping the person in such a way that it is not necessary for the reader to confront the uncomfortable reality that a unique person, with a particular set of friends and foes, strengths and weaknesses, fears and fantasies, pains and prejudices, has died in circumstances that are a painful reminder of our collective failure to provide for the disadvantaged.

As other chapters in this book describe, the stigma attached to mental illness may be as old as humanity itself and rooted in primitive and superstitious ideas of demonology. Stigmatizing attitudes are fed by stereotypes and maintained by ignorance, fear, and the tendency of public media to emphasize the sensational.

Stereotypes attached to the homeless are stigmatizing because they reflect a perception of failure in a success-oriented society, and implicit in the notion of failure is the notion of blameworthiness. Public attitudes to the homeless are often rejecting and unsympathetic (Marin 1988), and a backlash has been described in response to the ever-increasing numbers of beggars in city streets (Gibbs 1988). Common stigmatizing stereotypes of homeless persons are that they are dangerous, dishonest, dirty, lice-infested, drunken, unwilling to do honest work, and either relying shamelessly on public charity or rejecting proffered help.

Homeless mentally ill persons are thus doubly stigmatized. In addition to being subjected to the popular perceptions and misperceptions of the homeless, they are portrayed as the bizarre products of deinstitutionalization, discharged from the hospitals onto the streets. These generalizations, like all stereotypes, are oversimplified. Empirical research data, however, permit them to be examined and their aptness to be assessed.

The Baltimore Homeless Study

The Baltimore Homeless Study was designed to gather a comprehensive body of data on homeless people. The study examined not only the nature of their psychiatric disorders but also their place in society, as judged by their patterns of social relationships and contacts with social institutions. The data permit examination of the health and physical status of homeless people, their patterns of drug and alcohol use, their access to services, and the degree to which conflict with the norms of community behavior is manifested in frequent arrests and incarcerations (Breakey et al. 1989).

Methods

Data for the first stage of the study were collected in 1985–1986 from a random sample of 528 homeless people. Subjects were selected from among the residents of missions and shelters in Baltimore, Maryland, and from the Baltimore City Jail. A street survey was also conducted to determine how closely the sample selected could be assumed to resemble the total homeless population. Data from the street survey indicated that 75% of homeless people questioned on the street or outside a soup kitchen had been in one of the shelters or the jail within the preceding 6 months, so that they would have entered the sampling pool. A sampling plan was developed to obtain equal numbers of men and women over age 18, and subjects were interviewed with a survey instrument covering a wide variety of health and social history topics.

For the second stage, a subsample of 203 subjects was randomly selected to receive a comprehensive clinical evaluation. This protocol included a physical examination, laboratory tests, and an evaluation by a psychiatrist using the Standardized Psychiatric Examination (SPE) (Romanoski et al. 1988). The data resulting from the psychiatric examinations included detailed records of observed signs and symptoms, DSM-III (American Psychiatric Association 1980) diagnoses, and assessments of level of disability.

Men and women in the shelters and the jail and men in the missions constituted five strata for sampling and estimation. The numbers of persons in the strata on a typical night were estimated by making a census of missions and shelters (Breakey et al. 1986) and by projecting numbers of homeless people in the jail using data from jail rosters. Sampling within the five strata was not proportional to numbers in the strata, so weighted percentages were obtained by combining raw stratum percentages, weighted according to estimates of stratum size.

Findings

The data show that in general the subjects were very impaired in their health status and suffered many other disadvantages. Within this broad group of homeless people there was wide variation in many characteristics that did not necessarily conform to expectations.

Demographics. As noted in other studies of homeless people (e.g., Koegel et al. 1988; Roth et al. 1985; Susser et al. 1989), the ethnic composition of the sample showed an overrepresentation of minorities, approximately 62% of men and 71% of women (Table 10-1). Virtually all the minority subjects were black. For comparison, the population of the city of Baltimore is approximately 55% black (U.S. Department of Commerce 1980).

The subjects were predominantly in the young adult age group. Only 2% were over 65, contrasting with 13% in that age group in the general population. This bias toward younger age groups was particularly conspicuous in women, where one-fourth were below the age of 25. Among the men there was a substantial number, 36%, in the 45–64 year age group, conforming more closely to the traditional conception of a middle-aged homeless man.

Other characteristics. Several items from the baseline survey have been selected to illustrate some features of the population (see Tables 10-2 and 10-3). As a rule, the subjects were local people; 50% were born in the Baltimore area, and 80% had been in Baltimore for more than 6 months.

Their appearance was in most cases unexceptional. Evidence of lice or

Table 10–1. Race and sex distribution of randomly selected subjects from missions, shelters, and jail in the Baltimore Homeless Study

	Men ($n = 298$)	Women ($n = 230$)	Both sexes ($N = 528$)
Race			
White	37.9	29.2	35.3
Other races	62.1	70.8	64.7
Age (years)			
18–24	8.7	25.1	13.5
25–44	53.1	59.8	55.1
45–64	35.5	13.2	28.9
65 and above	2.0	1.9	2.0

Note. Rates, weighted across sites, in percent.

other infestations was detected by the interviewers in fewer than 2%. Bizarre or outlandish attire was also noted in only 2%. Dirty appearance or body odor was noted in 15% to 20% of men and approximately 5% of women.

The poverty of these individuals was extreme. Approximately one-half of subjects had incomes from all sources of less than $150 in the month prior to interview. In spite of their severe poverty, only 40% of men and 55% of women were receiving any type of public financial support. Only one in every three men or one in every two women said that public support was their main source of income. One-sixth were working, most in part-time jobs or casual labor, but 7% had full-time work.

When asked to describe their current health status, about half described it as "fair" to "poor." Almost one-fifth had been hospitalized for general health problems within the previous year. Half of the subjects obtained scores on the General Health Questionnaire (Goldberg 1972) that were indicative of significant levels of anxiety and depression.

In many cases these homeless people came from difficult backgrounds (Table 10-3). Twenty-eight percent had family histories of psychiatric disorder; approximately 50% had family histories of alcoholism. One in every five men and two in every five women gave histories of having been victims of child abuse. Their educational attainments were limited; only 40% had completed high school, compared with approximately 70% of the American

Table 10–2. Selected characteristics of homeless men and women in the Baltimore Homeless Study

	Men (n = 298)	Women (n = 230)	Both sexes (N = 528)
Permanence			
Born in Baltimore area	48.4	58.7	51.5
In Baltimore more than 6 months	76.8	85.1	79.3
Personal hygiene			
Outlandish dress	2.1	2.5	2.2
Dirty	15.2	5.8	12.4
Body odor	20.4	4.2	15.6
Lice	1.8	0	1.3
Income and employment			
Income less than $150 in past month	53.0	34.4	47.5
Working at least part-time	17.4	16.2	17.1
Receiving public funds	40.8	55.8	45.2
Public funds main source of income	33.9	53.5	39.7
Self-reported health status			
Health reported as "fair" to "poor"	48.0	47.7	47.9
GHQ score more than 4	47.5	57.4	50.4
Hospitalized past year	18.5	18.8	18.6

Note. Characteristics, weighted across sites, in percent. GHQ = General Health Questionnaire (Goldberg 1972).

population as a whole (U.S. Department of Health and Human Services 1986).

In general, homeless persons' current networks of relationships are fragile. One-third of men and one-fourth of women say they have no friends. However, the most striking findings are in relation to marital ties: only 4% were married at time of interview, in contrast to 49% of subjects in a Baltimore household sample (Kramer et al. 1987). The proportion of those never married (56.4%) was high in the homeless population, compared with the rate in households (26%), as was the proportion who were formerly married but now separated, widowed, or divorced (40% vs. 26% in house-

Table 10–3. Selected characteristics of homeless men and women in the Baltimore Homeless Study

	Men ($n = 298$)	Women ($n = 230$)	Both sexes ($N = 528$)
Early life			
Family history of mental disorder	24.8	36.3	28.2
Family history of alcohol problems	54.8	44.3	51.7
Family history of arrest	33.1	38.5	34.7
Abused as a child	19.9	40.1	25.9
High school graduate	38.6	44.7	40.4
Social networks			
Currently married	2.0	7.4	3.6
Formerly married	41.0	37.7	40.0
Never married	56.9	55.0	56.4
In contact with family	27.5	52.4	34.9
No friends at all	33.7	25.9	31.4
Victimization			
Victim of crime since homeless	36.8	17.5	31.1
Sexually assaulted within past year	0.2	4.2	1.4
Injury due to assault in past year	4.9	0.9	3.8
Arrests			
Ever arrested as juvenile	34.5	15.8	29.0
Ever arrested as adult	74.6	33.8	62.6
Ever convicted of felony	22.7	2.4	16.7

Note. Characteristics, weighted across sites, in percent.

holds). Only one in four men and one in two women were currently in touch with their families.

The alienation of homeless people is reflected in their involvement with antisocial activity, both as victims and as perpetrators. Approximately 37% of men and 18% of women said they had been victims of crime; 11 women (4.2%) and two men (0.2%) reported having been sexually assaulted in the past year. Three-fourths of men and one-third of women said they had been arrested at some time as adults, mostly for relatively minor offenses such as shoplifting or public nuisance offenses. However, there was also a significant proportion (17%) who had been convicted of felonies.

Psychiatric examinations.   A summary of the results of the psychiatrists' examinations is presented in Table 10-4. Overall, the percentage of people with DSM-III Axis I diagnoses was very high (89% of men and 74% of women). When substance use disorders were excluded, the rates were still as high as 60% for men and 70% for women. The Axis I prevalence rates

Table 10–4.   Psychiatric examination findings in the Baltimore Homeless Study

	Men (n = 125)	Women (n = 78)	Both sexes (N = 203)
Axis I			
Schizophrenia	8.3	15.7	10.5
Bipolar disorder	6.4	11.3	7.8
Major depression (unipolar)	13.8	14.0	13.9
Any major mental illness	33.8	46.8	37.7
Anxiety disorders (panic, obsessive-compulsive, generalized anxiety)	5.9	10.4	7.3
Adjustment disorders	5.4	8.4	6.3
Alcohol abuse/dependence	69.6	24.9	56.4
Other drug abuse/dependence	27.1	11.0	22.4
"Dual diagnosis" (mental illness and substance use disorder)	25.6	20.6	24.1
Any Axis I disorder	89.2	74.1	84.7
Axis II			
Paranoid personality	15.7	16.5	15.9
Schizoid personality	12.7	10.6	12.1
Antisocial personality	12.0	3.0	9.4
Avoidant personality	5.2	8.0	6.0
Any personality disorder	42.6	41.1	42.1
Mental retardation	4.4	5.2	4.6

Note.   Percent prevalence (including active cases and cases in remission) of selected DSM-III (American Psychiatric Association 1980) disorders, weighted across sites.

encompass a wide range of disorders of all levels of severity. For any major mental illness (e.g., schizophrenia, major affective disorders), the rates were 34% in men and 47% in women. Anxiety disorders (generalized anxiety, panic, and obsessive-compulsive disorders) were diagnosed in approximately 6% of men and 10% of women and adjustment disorders in 5% of men and 8% of women.

Substance abuse and dependence were extremely frequent. Alcohol abuse or dependence, either active or in remission, was noted in 70% of men and 25% of women. Two-thirds of these were currently active cases. The prevalence of other substance use disorders was also noteworthy, diagnosed in 27% of men and 11% of women. In many cases alcoholism and other substance abuse occurred along with other conditions, in particular the personality disorders. "Dual diagnosis" was common: approximately 26% of

Table 10–5. Psychiatric hospitalization history of examined subjects, mentally ill and not mentally ill, in the Baltimore Homeless Study

| | Psychiatric hospitalization | | |
	Ever admitted	Never admitted	n
Mentally ill subjects	52.9	47.1	85
Not mentally ill	13.8	86.2	116
All examined subjects	30.3	69.7	201
	Number of psychiatric admissions		
	0–3	More than 3	n
Mentally ill subjects	77.2	22.8	79
Not mentally ill	98.2	1.8	112
All examined subjects	89.5	10.5	181
	Longest episode of inpatient care*		
	Up to 3 mos.	More than 3 mos.	n
Mentally ill subjects	52.6	47.4	38
Not mentally ill	92.9	7.1	14
All examined subjects	63.5	36.5	52

Note. Unweighted data; rates percent.
*Of those ever admitted.

Table 10–6. Current functional status of mentally ill subjects in the Baltimore Homeless Study

| | n | Current level of social and occupational functioning | |
		% of mentally ill subjects ($n = 84$)	% of all examined subjects ($N = 200$)
DSM-III Axis V			
1–3 (Superior-Good)	3	3.6	1.5
4–5 (Fair-Poor)	51	60.7	25.5
6–7 (Severely impaired)	28	33.3	14.0

Note. Unweighted data.

men and 21% of women were diagnosed with both a major mental illness and a substance use disorder.

Personality disorders were diagnosed in approximately 40% of men and women. The paranoid, schizoid, avoidant, and, in men, antisocial personality types were most often diagnosed. Mental retardation was diagnosed, on clinical criteria, in approximately 5% of men and women.

Finally, an attempt was made to give an estimate of how many mentally ill subjects might be considered "severely" mentally ill, conforming to the public stereotype of the deinstitutionalized patient who is severely dysfunctional and discharged from hospital after a long period of inpatient care. Tables 10-5 and 10-6 display data relating to hospitalization history and level of functioning. Only one-half of those with major mental illnesses admitted having been a psychiatric inpatient at any time. Approximately 23% had been admitted more than three times. Of those who had been admitted at any time, only half had been admitted for a period of 3 months or more. In other words, although 30% of the total sample had been admitted at some time, only 10% of the sample were mentally ill persons who had been admitted more than three times, and a similar proportion were mentally ill persons who had been admitted at some time for a period of 3 months or more.

As another measure of severity, an estimate of current level of functioning was made for each subject by the examining psychiatrist, using Axis V of DSM-III (American Psychiatric Association 1980). By this measure, one-

Table 10–7. Frequency of selected physical health problems in examined subjects in the Baltimore Homeless Study

	Men ($n = 120$)	Women ($n = 75$)
Oral and dental	67.5	65.3
Gynecological		64.0
Dermatological	57.5	56.0
Cardiovascular	52.5	46.7
Musculoskeletal	37.5	45.3
Respiratory	40.0	40.0
Neurological	33.3	37.3
Anemia	18.3	34.7
Sexually transmitted disease	7.5	10.7
Average number of problems per subject	8.3	9.2

Note. Data, unweighted, in percent.

third of the mentally ill subjects were noted to be severely impaired (i.e., their level of functioning was rated to be "very poor" or "grossly impaired"). Thus 14% of the total examined sample were mentally ill and severely impaired in functional capacity (Table 10-6).

Physical findings. In addition to the wide range of psychopathology found in the psychiatric examinations, physical examinations revealed that this group of people suffered from many physical problems (Table 10-7). These problems included those common in any group of people, such as hypertension or prostatic enlargement, but also an overrepresentation of conditions associated with the homeless life-style, poor nutrition, alcohol abuse, and lack of basic primary health care (Stine et al. 1988).

Discussion

These data provide an opportunity to evaluate some of the assumptions that underlie stigmatizing attitudes toward homeless mentally ill people. To some extent the stereotypes contain a kernel of truth; for the most part, they are wide of the mark.

One common allegation in many cities is that these are transients, people from "out of town," or "just passing through," who are "taking advantage of the services provided in the city." These data show that the majority of homeless people in Baltimore are Baltimoreans; at least half were born in the area, and almost all have been in Baltimore for more than 6 months.

The common view that most homeless people are dirty, bizarrely dressed, unkempt, and infested with lice or other parasites was also shown to be untrue. In more than 80% of cases, there was nothing unusual about the appearance or personal hygiene of these subjects. Indeed, maintaining such a good level of external appearances must require considerable motivation, and at times ingenuity, in light of the poor facilities available to most homeless people.

Myths that circulate about homeless people amassing money that they refuse to spend for their own basic needs are also shown to be highly unlikely. The average income of these persons was less than $5 per day. The other notion—that they parasitically live off the public purse—is also shown to be untrue: fewer than half of them were receiving any public entitlements.

In general, their health was poor, by their own estimate and as judged on the basis of careful clinical assessment. On the General Health Questionnaire, a measure of general distress and malaise, the proportion scoring above the usual cut-off was about four times that in the general population. Homeless people as a group are, undoubtedly, more subject to the diseases that occur under conditions of harsh environment, limited opportunity for practicing good personal hygiene, and poor nutrition (Breakey et al. 1989; Gelberg and Linn 1989; Wright and Weber 1987).

The reality, as shown by these data, is that homeless people are truly on the fringe of society. They often come from families with major problems, were often abused as children, and, in 60% of the cases, did not graduate from high school. Their alienation is reflected in the fragmented nature of their networks of relationships, their lack of marital ties, their victimization, and their frequent confrontations with the police.

One of the most enduring stigmatizing stereotypes of the homeless person is that of the alcoholic, the "skid-row bum," or "wino": the older male, dirty, disheveled and deteriorated. Both alcoholism and drug abuse are strongly disapproved of in our culture, with their connotations of poor self-control and socially deteriorated behavior. Data from this study are consistent with reports from others (Fischer 1989; Mulkern and Spence 1984) demonstrating the very high frequency of alcoholism among homeless people of both sexes, in all age groups. Most homeless alcoholic individuals do not conform to the "skid row" stereotype, but the alcoholism has nonetheless taken a severe toll upon their social functioning and physical health (Koegel and Burnam 1988; Stine et al. 1988).

In spite of the persisting high prevalence of substance use disorders, the alcoholic stereotype has largely been replaced in the public mind by that of the deinstitutionalized mental patient. However, this stereotype has only limited validity. Although the prevalence of mental illness is many times higher than in the general population, the data suggest that only a minority

meet the criterion of "severely" mentally ill. Only about one homeless
person in seven can be characterized as both mentally ill and severely
impaired. It is commonly stated that one-third of the homeless have histories of mental hospitalization, with the implication that this indicates significant mental disability. In this sample, too, almost one-third had been in
a psychiatric hospital at some time, but not all of these subjects had been
diagnosed by the psychiatrists as mentally ill. What is more, only 10% of the
subjects admitted having had a period of psychiatric inpatient treatment in
excess of 3 months. The notion that everyone who has been in a psychiatric
hospital should be considered severely mentally ill represents another form
of stereotyping.

Apart from any consideration of psychiatric disorder, homeless people in
general are regarded as being of poor character, failures, who have become
unemployed and lack the qualities needed to succeed. Their precarious life
and downward social mobility are contrary to what is esteemed in people,
and they are all the more despised because of the common belief that they
choose to live this way. Objective and comprehensive assessment of character is complex. This study relied upon the assessments of experienced psychiatrists and the use of several standard scales. Antisocial traits were noted
in a proportion, to be sure, and the subjects' arrest records demonstrate that
many get involved in antisocial acts. An associated study, however, has
shown that many of the offenses committed by homeless people are in the
nature of survival crimes, such as shoplifting food articles or entering a
boarded-up house to seek shelter; others are related to drunkenness or the
public consumption of alcohol (Fischer 1988). In terms of personality, however, it is important to note that schizoid, schizotypal, and paranoid traits
are more common than antisocial traits. These traits contribute to patterns
of isolation, anxiety, and timidity that are most characteristic of the homeless population, leading many to describe themselves as "loners" and increasing their vulnerability to homelessness.

This analysis shows that many common opinions about homeless people
are not supported by data. They are opinions, nevertheless, that are often
strongly held and thus contribute to negative public perceptions of homeless
people in general and the homeless mentally ill in particular. In addition, the
homeless population has certain group characteristics that are unjustly
subject to public disapproval in a success-oriented society: they are the
poorest of the poor, and a sizeable majority are unemployed. In a society in
which racism is still an active social force, ethnic minorities are overrepre-
sented. Whether based on fantasy or fact, stigma serves to increase the
distancing of a group of people who are already predisposed by their character and their illnesses to be isolated and to have low self-esteem.

The homeless mentally ill, therefore, experience compounded disadvantages. Some shelters are reluctant to admit them. Mentally ill people,

well aware of this prejudice, will often attempt to conceal their psychiatric histories or shun potential havens from the street. In the eyes of many in the general community, also, they are viewed with disdain, increasing their difficulty in being accepted and depriving them of the social supports that might enable them to maintain a residence, even in difficult times.

Responses to Homeless Mentally Ill Persons

Stigmatizing attitudes toward homeless mentally ill persons have their impact at the level of individual conduct and in the formulation of public policy. To minimize these effects, a number of steps would be likely to help in modifying public perceptions.

Stigma is fostered by ignorance and built upon a foundation of stereotypes. More than anything else, the development and dissemination of sound knowledge about mental illness and homelessness will reduce stereotyping and prejudice. Good public information, based on sound scholarship, is a first requisite for dispelling myths. Discussions of the homeless should emphasize their diversity to combat the creation and persistence of stereotypes. It should be constantly emphasized that homelessness is an endpoint at which a wide variety of people arrive for a wide variety of reasons. It is vital to draw attention to the adverse circumstances facing very poor people in our society and to emphasize that it is these economic and social pressures that cause vulnerable people to become homeless.

Every effort should be made to educate the public that alcoholism is a health problem rather than to be dismissed as a sign of moral degeneracy, and that public health measures, rather than condemnation of the victims, are the appropriate response. The high prevalence of psychiatric and substance use disorders does not justify casting blame; rather, it provides a challenge to psychiatrists and other service providers to do better in meeting the varied treatment needs of the addicted and the mentally ill. Accessible and acceptable health and other services should be provided in such a way that homeless people can get help with those conditions that serve to increase stigma and prevent resettlement. Making such people welcome in mainstream service systems also will serve to lessen the stigmatization that may be an inadvertent consequence of the segregation of these people into special programs.

Efforts to help homeless people, as is true for mentally ill persons, succeed best when they focus upon the restoration of morale. It is important to treat homeless people with dignity and to enhance their self-esteem. As much as anyone, they deserve safe and pleasant surroundings. Dirty, primitive, overcrowded shelters, miserable hotel accommodations, or the massive warehouses that are to be found in major cities may provide crude shelter from the elements, but they do nothing to help a man or woman escape from the cycle of homelessness. These institutions may, indeed, demoralize their inmates and foster the culture of homelessness in such a way that escape becomes more difficult. Some of the most successful programs focus upon the capacity of their participants to take an active, rather than passive, role in organizing the program and delivering the service.

Conclusion

Many of the stereotypes of homelessness that are common in our culture have little basis in fact. Like all stereotypes, they are oversimplifications; they tend to exaggerate certain characteristics and fail to describe the great variety of people within the homeless population. In particular, the "severely mentally ill" stereotype can only be applied to a small proportion of today's homeless people. Stereotypes are stigmatizing, and the added burden of negative perceptions suffered by the homeless and the mentally ill persons can only make it more difficult for them to escape from their miserable situation.

The question remains to be addressed as to whether psychiatrists and psychiatric epidemiologists are guilty of increasing stigma or provide an opportunity for "blaming the victim" when they emphasize the psychiatric disorders and substance abuse problems of homeless people, or whether "cold statistics" (Hilfiker 1989) have a depersonalizing effect in consideration of this heart-wrenching human problem. Instead of using empirical data such as these to demonstrate the neediness of homeless people and as ammunition in the struggle to obtain better services, advocates often choose to deemphasize the role of substance abuse and mental illness, focusing instead upon the economic and social causes of homelessness. Psychiatrists are sometimes thought to be insulting the homeless and distracting public attention from problems such as poverty and the lack of affordable housing that underlie their present dilemma.

It is certainly true that those unsympathetic to the homeless population can use research findings against them ("The Ill Homeless" 1989). The fact that mental illness and substance abuse still bear a great burden of stigma is not sufficient reason, however, to deny their importance among homeless people. Rather, it is incumbent upon advocates for the people who are homeless to join forces with their colleagues in advocacy for those who are mentally ill to combat stereotyping and stigmatizing attitudes at every level in the society in which they are to be found. Apart from all other considerations, homelessness is all the more scandalous because it is the most vulnerable among us who are disproportionately affected.

References

American Psychiatric Association: Diagnostic and Statistical Manual of Mental Disorders, 3rd Edition. Washington, DC, American Psychiatric Association, 1980

Breakey WR, Fischer PJ, Cowan CD: Homeless people in Baltimore: demographic profile and enumeration. Paper presented at the annual meeting of the American Public Health Association, Las Vegas, NV, Sept 1986

Breakey WR, Fischer PJ, Kramer M, et al: Health and mental health problems of homeless men and women in Baltimore. JAMA 262:1352–1357, 1989

Fischer PJ: Criminal activity among the homeless: a study of arrests in Baltimore. Hosp Community Psychiatry 9:46–51, 1988

Fischer PJ: Estimating prevalence of alcohol, drug and mental health problems in the contemporary homeless population: a review of the literature. Contemporary Drug Problems 16:333–389, 1989

Gelberg L, Linn LS: Assessing the physical health of homeless adults. JAMA 262:1973–1979, 1989

Gibbs NR: Begging: to give or not to give. Time, Sept 5, 1988

Goldberg DP: The Detection of Mental Illness by Questionnaire. London, Oxford University Press, 1972

Hilfiker D: Are we comfortable with homelessness? JAMA 262:1375–1376, 1989

The ill homeless. Wall Street Journal, Oct 6, 1989

Koegel P, Burnam A: Alcoholism among homeless adults in the inner city of Los Angeles. Arch Gen Psychiatry 45:1011–1018, 1988

Koegel P, Burnam A, Farr RK: The prevalence of specific psychiatric disorders among homeless individuals in the inner city of Los Angeles. Arch Gen Psychiatry 45:1085–1092, 1988

Kramer M, Brown H, Skinner A, et al: Changing living arrangements in the population and their potential effect on the prevalence of mental disorder: findings of the Eastern Baltimore Mental Health Survey, in Psychiatric Epidemiology: Progress and Prospects. Edited by Cooper B. London, Croom & Helm, 1987, pp 3–26

Marin P: Helping and hating the homeless. Harpers, Jan 1988, pp 39–49

Mulkern V, Spence R: Alcohol abuse/alcoholism among homeless persons: a review of the literature. Rockville, MD, National Institute on Alcoholism and Alcohol Abuse, 1984

Romanoski AR, Nestadt G, Chahal R, et al: Inter-observer reliability of a "Standardized Psychiatric Examination" (SPE) for case ascertainment (DSM III). J Nerv Ment Dis 176:63–71, 1988

Roth D, Bean J, Lust N, et al: Homelessness in Ohio: A Study of People in Need. Columbus, OH, Ohio Department of Mental Health, 1985

Stine OC, Fischer PJ, Breakey WR: Co-morbid physical problems of homeless mentally ill persons in Baltimore. Paper presented at the 116th annual meeting of the American Public Health Association, Boston, MA, Nov 1988

Susser E, Struening EL, Conover S: Psychiatric problems in homeless men. Arch Gen Psychiatry 46:845–850, 1989

U.S. Department of Commerce, Bureau of the Census: General Population Characteristics: Maryland. Washington, DC, U.S. Department of Commerce, 1980

U.S. Department of Health and Human Services: Health Status of the Disadvantaged: Chartbook 1968. (DHHS No. [HRSA] HRS-P-DV86-2). Washington, DC, U.S. Department of Health and Human Services, 1986

Wright JD, Weber E: Homelessness and Health. Washington, DC, McGraw-Hill, 1987

Chapter 11

Cinematic Stereotypes Contributing to the Stigmatization of Psychiatrists

Glen O. Gabbard, M.D.
Krin Gabbard, Ph.D.

Stigmatization of mentally ill persons is obvious in our society. What is less immediately obvious is the stigmatization of psychiatrists who treat mental illness. However, prejudice and stereotyping of psychiatrists are entrenched aspects of American culture. Gabbard and Gabbard investigate some cinematic stereotypes of psychiatrists that reflect this prejudice and stereotyping.

An analysis of the psychiatric role in many films reveals both good and bad stereotypical images of psychiatrists. The authors examine the ways in which these images and distortions affect patients, and the deterrent effect on medical students considering a career in psychiatry.

They conclude that psychiatrists must accept that "their roles as transference objects transcend the confines of the consulting room and spread onto the great silver screen."

The stigmatization of psychiatrists is a complex phenomenon that derives from multiple sources. Long before most people have actually met a psychiatrist, they have been bombarded with numerous images of mental health professionals in movies and television, not to mention media as diverse as magazine cartoons and the patter of nightclub comedians. If we confine ourselves to theatrically released American movies, we find that from 1906 through 1989 there are at least 300 films featuring a psychiatrist or other mental health professional. These myriad celluloid depictions are not irrelevant to the public's understanding of psychiatric treatment. As we shall demonstrate, the cinema in this country has been a major contributor to the stigmatization of psychiatrists.

The cinema generates a multitude of images that reflect our time and that touch on fundamental human psychological processes with which psychiatrists and patients alike identify. For contemporary audiences, attending movies is an experience that provides catharsis and unites the audience with their culture in much the same way that the tragedies of Sophocles and Aeschylus performed these functions for 5th-century B.C. Greek audiences. Cinematic portrayals of various professional groups serve to construct a cultural mythology that becomes a part of the collective unconscious of the American public.

In *Psychiatry and the Cinema* (Gabbard and Gabbard 1987) we were able to trace historically the rise and fall of the cinematic image of the psychiatrist. The early years between 1906 and 1957 present a bifurcated myth of psychiatry. On the one hand there are an assortment of alienists, mesmerists, and buffoons of questionable training and expertise, often equipped with thick Viennese accents, pince-nez, goatees, and inscrutable jargon. On the other hand, the war years brought more positive depictions of impressive psychotherapists who were able to make bedridden soldiers walk and who could solve crimes that defied police investigation.

Between 1957 and 1963 we were able to identify a brief Golden Age of psychiatry in the cinema characterized by almost consistently idealized portraits of psychiatrists as compassionate and effective clinicians or oracular sleuths. From 1963 to 1980 we noted a fall from grace in which the psychiatrist was likely to be viewed again as a buffoon, an agent of a repressive society, a sadist who uses electroconvulsive therapy to retaliate against rebellious patients, or even a homicidal transvestite. The decade of the 1980s has been characterized by a mixed view of the profession, with many familiar stereotypes, but also some reconciliation to the notion that therapists are human, too.

Throughout each of these historical periods, skeptical attitudes about psychiatrists abound. As early as 1919 Victor Fleming directed *When the Clouds Roll By*, in which Herbert Grimwood plays a mysterious "doctor of the mind." When he is first introduced lecturing to an audience of his colleagues, a title card reads, "Here he confirms the popular prejudice of the time against the mushroom growth of dubious psychologists."

Schneider (1977, 1987) has categorized the cinematic stereotypes of psychiatrists into three groups represented by three stereotypes: Dr. Dippy, Dr. Evil, and Dr. Wonderful. Here we will subdivide the profession even further by delineating 10 cinematic stereotypes that can be found in virtually every historical period of the American cinema. We will discuss each of the 10 stereotypes and consider the contributions of these stereotypes to the stigmatization of mental health professionals.

Ten Cinematic Stereotypes of the Psychiatrist

The Libidinous Lecher

One legacy of psychoanalysis and the writings of Sigmund Freud is the association in the public's mind of psychiatry with sexuality. Through misunderstandings of Freud, a myth has developed that psychiatrists are primarily interested in sex and that the main thrust of psychiatric treatment is to awaken repressed sexuality in patients. Beginning with the first loosenings of the Production Code in the 1950s, the film industry found that psychiatrists could legitimize sexuality in films. Before the new ratings' system provided an atmosphere of sexual permissiveness in 1968, a number of films appeared with titles like *Three Nuts in Search of a Bolt*, *Suburbia Confidential*, *The Twisted Sex*, and even *Loves of a Psychiatrist*. These films were part of a rash of "nudies" that used psychiatry both to facilitate sex scenes and to give the film "redeeming social value." Not surprisingly, psychiatry lost much of its value to the adult film industry when the Supreme Court removed social redemption from its test for pornography.

At any rate, a well-established stereotype in the movies is the psychiatrist as seducer. There are evil versions of the seducer, such as Tom Conway in *The Cat People* (1942), and comical versions exemplified by Richard Benjamin in *Love at First Bite* (1979) and by Peter Sellers in *What's New Pussycat?* (1965). The seductive therapist is not always male in the movies. Colleen Dewhurst attempts to seduce Sean Connery in *A Fine Madness* (1966), and Natalie Wood is overtly seductive toward Tony Curtis in *Sex and the Single Girl* (1963).

The Eccentric Buffoon

Far and away the most common cinematic stereotype of psychiatrists is the eccentric buffoon. This version draws on the well-known myth that psychiatrists are crazier than their patients. Psychiatrists are often depicted with odd mannerisms and facial tics. Their pomposity is usually manifested by spouting obfuscating jargon. In Howard Hawks' *Bringing Up Baby* (1938), Fritz Feld presents a classic example of this stereotype when he distorts his face in a grotesque grimace after telling Katherine Hepburn that "all people who act strangely are not crazy."

In the 1930s, one variant of the eccentric buffoon was the Viennese-accented "expert" who was brought in to make definitive diagnoses or pronouncements of one variety or another, only to be proved wrong. In *Mr. Deeds Goes to Town* (1936), Frank Capra cast Wyrley Birch as Emile von Haller, "the most eminent psychiatrist in the world." Von Haller testifies in court that Mr. Deeds, played by Gary Cooper, is manic-depressive. Von Haller's credibility, however, is destroyed when Deeds points out that the

Viennese crackpot is given to childish doodling. In this film, as in many others, the psychiatrist is contrasted with "the common man." He is shown to lack common sense and to be completely irrelevant to the needs of the American people. He is often juxtaposed with actors like Cooper and Jimmy Stewart, whose mere presence on screen suggests small-town values of close-knit family, community involvement, friendly neighbors, and common sense. Adherence to these values, these films imply, is all that is required for mental health. Psychiatry is irrelevant.

The stereotype of the eccentric buffoon is by no means limited to the 1930s. The first psychiatrist in American film, the asylum director in *Dr. Dippy's Sanitarium* (1906), certainly fit that mold. Films of the 1980s are replete with such images. One scene in *Oh God! Book II* (1980) displays a whole room full of psychiatrists with nervous tics and other affectations. And Woody Allen films, of course, regularly exploit this stereotype.

The Unempathic Cold Fish

This stereotype probably stems from misunderstandings of psychoanalytic neutrality. Psychotherapists are regularly depicted in film as stonefaced, insensitive, uncaring, and ineffectual. In *The Deer Hunter* (1978), Christopher Walken's tears and distress are met with a blank expression by a military psychiatrist. In *Bob and Carol and Ted and Alice* (1969), directed by Paul Mazursky, real-life psychiatrist Donald Muhich stares blindly at Dyan Cannon as she struggles with her marital relationship, and he ushers her out the door while she is clearly in a state of turmoil. Muhich began as Paul Mazursky's psychiatrist, and since *Bob and Carol and Ted and Alice*, he has appeared in three other Mazursky films as a psychiatrist, most recently as the dog psychiatrist, unquestionably an eccentric buffoon, in *Down and Out in Beverly Hills* (1986).

The Rationalist Foil

A favorite depiction of science fiction and horror genres, this figure attempts to reduce the mysteries of supernatural events to psychodynamic formulations—only to be proved wrong. The scrupulously rational and earthbound work of psychiatrists provides the perfect foil for the generic conceit of the unknown, the unseen, and the unimagined. These psychiatrists often pay with their lives for their foolish adherence to the rational principles of scientific thought. Many of them are buffoonlike, such as the psychiatrist in *Poltergeist III* (1988) who attempts to convince his young patient that her otherworld visitors are merely a product of her imagination. After he and several colleagues witness a ghoulish hand appearing out of nowhere and hurling a coffee mug into a one-way mirror, the skeptical psychiatrist dismisses the entire incident as an example of "mass hypnosis."

While many rationalist foils are clearly buffoonlike as well, others are portrayed quite realistically. In *The Entity* (1983), Ron Silver plays a dedicated psychiatrist trying to help Barbara Hershey. He is shown to be sensitive, empathic, and astute. However, he is not sharp enough to realize that all of his patient's problems are due to an invisible demon rapist.

Walt Disney films, such as *The Gnomemobile* and *The Shaggy Dog*, have also used the rationalist foil. When Tommy Kirk turns into a dog in the latter film, his father (played by Fred McMurray) seeks psychiatric consultation. He is told that his son's canine transformation is a product of his own imagination, representing his "submerged second self."

The Repressive Agent of Society

Part of the irony of the stigmatizing cinematic images associated with psychiatry is that often diametrically opposed stereotypes coexist. For example, one common view of psychiatrists is that they are akin to witch doctors who unleash powerful sexual forces from the chains of repression. Equally common, however, is the view that psychiatrists are repressive agents of society who intimidate their patients into submitting to the constricting values of the society.

Although this version of the film psychiatrist can be found throughout the history of American film, it is perhaps most pronounced in the latter 1960s and early 1970s, when Hollywood appropriated the counterculture's view that psychiatry was a tool of the establishment to force conformity on creative free spirits. According to the mythology attached to this stereotype, mental health professionals badger patients into accepting society's values rather than changing them. In *Harold and Maude* (1971), director Hal Ashby places psychiatry in a class with the military and organized religion as one of the major establishment forces in the society. Teenager Harold (played by Bud Cort) is in love with octogenarian Maude (Ruth Gordon), much to his mother's chagrin. To deal with his aberrant tastes, his mother sends him to three different authority figures: a military officer, a psychiatrist, and a priest. Each admonishes him about the perils of deviating from culturally sanctioned choices of appropriate romantic partners.

When the patient is female and the psychiatrist male, psychotherapy is frequently depicted as a forum in which the therapist attempts to persuade his patient to submit to male domination instead of trying to assert herself as an independent person, as in *Diary of a Mad Housewife* (1970). The reverse situation is depicted in *One Flew Over the Cuckoo's Nest* (1975), in which a female professional, Nurse Ratched (played by Louise Fletcher), demands that her passive male patients submit to her domination. The Jack Nicholson character is portrayed as a free spirit and liberator of the tyrannized patients. His punishment for challenging the authority of Nurse Ratched is lobotomy.

The Unfulfilled Woman

While most cinematic stereotypes are applicable to both genders, there is at least one stereotype that appears to belong exclusively to the female practitioner. Whenever a woman psychiatrist treats a male patient, she is almost invariably portrayed as an unfulfilled single woman who works compulsively to make up for a lack of fulfillment in her personal life. The woman psychiatrist is usually "cured" by the love of a male patient, who turns tables on her by demonstrating to her that *she* is the one in need of help. The love of the male patient brings these women to life so that they no longer need their careers. A perfect example of this stereotype is found in the 1954 Danny Kaye movie *Knock on Wood*. Kaye plays a ventriloquist who seeks analytic treatment after his dummy repeatedly expresses split-off and disavowed feelings of the ventriloquist toward his girlfriends. Shortly after beginning the treatment, however, Danny Kaye makes it eminently clear that his analyst, played by Mai Zetterling, is far more in need of *his* help than he is in need of *hers*. After a cursory reading of Freud, he explains to his analyst that she is suffering from survivor guilt in reaction to her fiance's death. She responds with insight and abreaction to her patient's interpretation and ultimately decides to marry him.

We have been able to identify at least 20 American films that conform to this stereotype and have devoted an entire paper to the subject (see Gabbard and Gabbard 1989). While it might be tempting to dismiss this depiction as a product of the prefeminist historical era, 6 of these 20 films are products of the 1980s.

The Evil Mind Doctor

This stereotype, a variant of the traditional "mad scientist," goes back at least to 1919, when Herbert Grimwood unscrupulously attempted to drive Douglas Fairbanks to suicide in *When the Clouds Roll By*. In this tradition psychiatry is merely a front for criminal activity. These therapists blackmail their patients, manipulate them, murder them, and otherwise exploit them for their own gain. For example, in *Nightmare Alley* (1947), Helen Walker plays Lilith Ritter, a "counseling psychologist" who is sought out by Stanton Carlisle, a nightclub "mentalist" played by Tyrone Power. Dr. Ritter enlists her patient's help in an elaborate scheme for extorting money from wealthy patients who are obsessed with deceased loved ones. After conspiring to divest one wealthy patient of $150,000, Dr. Ritter has no further use for her patient. When he threatens to expose her, she begins speaking in the patronizing tones of a therapist, suggesting that he is mentally unstable. When he hears police sirens, she informs him that he must be hallucinating.

The Vindictive Psychiatrist

Psychiatrists spend years of training and supervision learning to harness their emotional reactions to patients, usually referred to as *counter-transference*. They are taught to reflect on these feelings as important sources of information about themselves and their patients rather than to act on them. Filmmakers, however, have responded to widely publicized reports of therapists who abuse patients by regularly suggesting that psychiatrists act out intense countertransference feelings, whether they be sexual or aggressive in nature. The vindictive psychiatrist employs psychiatric treatments as retaliation or punishment growing out of powerful emotional reactions evoked by the patient. In *Frances* (1982), insulin shock is portrayed as a punishment inflicted on Frances (played by Jessica Lange) for her contemptuous behavior toward her psychiatrist. As mentioned above, treatment as retaliation is also part of *One Flew Over the Cuckoo's Nest* (1975). In *St. Ives* (1975), the vindictive psychiatrist stereotype reaches the ultimate caricature. Without question this film deserves inclusion in any compendium of "Great Moments in the Countertransference." Dr. John Constable (played by Maximillian Schell) is the live-in psychiatrist for millionaire Abner Procane (played by John Houseman). After he becomes fed up with his patient's neurosis, Dr. Constable plots to deprive him of his fortune. His countertransference erupts when he produces a gun and shoots Procane after professing his hatred of him. The absurdity of this depiction is challenged only by *Dressed to Kill*, the 1980 film in which Michael Caine dresses as a woman and murders female patients who arouse him sexually.

The Omniscient Detective

The image of the psychotherapist as a sleuth pursuing and solving the mysteries of the unconscious mind has been appropriated by Hollywood for use in the crime genre. Numerous films in the 1940s, including *Conflict* (1945), *Crime Doctor* (1943), and *Dark Waters* (1944), portray mental health professionals as detectives who are superior to police in their crime-solving capacities because of their ability to see into the unconscious mind of the criminal. A prime example of the confusion between the psychiatrist and the detective can be found in the last scene of *Psycho* (1960), in which Simon Oakland portrays a forensic psychiatrist. The brilliant psychoanalytic formulation provided by the psychiatrist after conducting a brief forensic evaluation of the murderer would inspire envy and awe in every psychiatrist who has ever consulted with a police department or a prison. One might question why such an idealized portrayal of psychiatry is included in a discussion of stigma. Certain positive portrayals of mental health professionals can be just as stigmatizing as negative portrayals in that they misrepresent psychiatry to the public and mislead patients into expecting the impossible.

The Dramatic Healer

Another idealized portrayal of psychiatry that is stigmatizing is the dramatic healer. A recurrent aspect of the "talking cure" depicted in films about psychotherapy is the cathartic cure. In these films a psychiatrist dramatically uncovers a repressed traumatic memory that seems to cure the patient instantly. These fanciful portrayals of cure mislead potential patients into expecting dramatic and greatly oversimplified cures from their therapists. As Schneider (1987) notes, this flow of cure reflects a more general trend in movie psychiatry to operate on its own peculiar set of principles that bear only a faint resemblance to those of real-life psychiatry. In the "Golden Age" movie *The Three Faces of Eve* (1957), a psychiatrist (played by Lee J. Cobb) hypnotizes Eve (played by Joanne Woodward) and helps her recall a repressed traumatic memory of being forced to kiss her dead grandmother. The film suggests that the recall of this memory completely cures her of multiple personality disorder. Her three personalities are spontaneously integrated into one.

This depiction of psychiatric cure is pure myth. In her 1977 autobiography, the real-life Eve, Chris Costner Sizemore, revealed that in fact the recovery of the repressed traumatic memory did not lead to a lasting resolution of her multiple personalities. Following the treatment represented in the film, more personalities appeared, a total of 22 in all. She finally attained what she considered to be a lasting recovery in 1974 following a suicide attempt and more intensive therapy.

The cathartic cure may be psychiatric myth, but it is good drama. Obviously, the "showbiz" value of any treatment is of much more importance to filmmakers than its clinical accuracy. It is of interest in this regard that the effective prescribing of psychotropic medication and its role in treatment are virtually unheard of in American film. Psychiatric treatment is almost always depicted as psychotherapy. Notable exceptions, of course, are barbaric depictions of electroconvulsive therapy in films such as *The Snake Pit* (1948), *Shock Corridor* (1963), and *One Flew Over the Cuckoo's Nest* (1975). But it is clear that the biological revolution in psychiatry has yet to reach the screen.

Contributions to Stigma

In considering the contribution of these stereotypes to stigma, a good place to start is the following question: Are they distortions? The omniscient detective and the dramatic healer are certainly out of keeping with what we know of typical clinical practice. But what about the more negative depictions? Surveys of psychiatrists, psychologists, and social workers document that a small but significant percentage of practitioners have engaged in sexual relations with patients (Gabbard 1989). There are certainly well-known reports of abuses of electroconvulsive therapy and psychosurgery in public hospitals. So are these depictions distortions? Yes and no. They are *not* distortions in the sense that a handful of psychiatrists essentially fit the cinematic stereotypes. On the other hand, these portrayals *are* distortions in the sense that they do not accurately represent the typical, modal, well-intentioned psychiatrist, who attempts to master countertransference feelings in the service of delivering humane and effective psychiatric care.

The problem with this distinction, however, is that a naive audience member may or may not have any familiarity with psychiatrists outside the movie theater and may therefore be completely in the dark regarding the customary behavior of a typical psychiatrist. Uninformed audience members may have no standard by which to judge the appropriateness and the frequency of what they witness on the screen. Returning to the comparison of modern movie audiences with ancient Greek theatergoers, like tragic heroes, film characters may be viewed as archetypes who represent the entire profession. Their core characteristics may be assumed to qualify them as a kind of psychiatric Everyman, leading the naive audience member to think, "So that is what psychiatrists are like" (Gabbard and Gabbard 1987).

Because no two psychiatrists would probably agree on which cinematic portrayals are the most accurate, it may be of more heuristic value to view the film psychiatrist as a transference object. The psychiatrist, whether in movies or in real life, is perhaps particularly subject to transference distortions. As Paul Fink (1983) has pointed out:

> While all physicians have their roots in the priesthood and in the rights of the society, they do not retain the mantle of magic incantation as do psychiatrists. Aesculapian authority has evolved in a nonverbal direction. Psychiatry is often called upon to deal with mental pain such as guilt (which is more akin to priestly authority than Aesculapian authority). (p. 673)

Psychiatrists may be more vulnerable to significant transferential distortions because they can so easily be regarded as omniscient mind readers who understand the dark workings of the human psyche in a manner unavailable to others. Indeed, it is this dimension that is often depicted in movies about psychiatrists. These powers are frightening, and people may make fun of them in order to deal with the anxiety aroused by them.

Psychiatrists must take the blame for some of these distortions as well. Historically, psychiatry has contributed to its own mystification by encouraging the perception that it contains answers to all questions and by promising remedies for highly complex social problems that are well beyond its purview (Fink 1983). Moreover, the use of obfuscating jargon by so many eccentric buffoons in the cinema did not grow out of a vacuum. Psychiatrists have enhanced the trend toward mystification by talking and writing in a tongue that is as unfamiliar as a foreign language to most outsiders.

The core question involving stigmatization, however, involves the impact of these stereotypes on patients or potential patients. Some psychiatrists are highly skeptical that cinematic images seriously influence a person's attitude toward his or her current or future therapist. Any intelligent patient, the argument goes, can discriminate between the celluloid portrayal and the "real McCoy." This argument paints the moviegoer as a purely rational thinker beyond the influence of unconscious forces. Media images work on us unconsciously throughout our lives, even if we consciously reject the film stereotypes that we see. We all harbor a mental warehouse full of internal stereotypes coded in preconscious and unconscious memory banks. The crooked politician, the heroic warrior, the whore with a heart of gold, and the socially inept intellectual are all examples of such internal stereotypes. Madison Avenue has mined these subliminally perceived and stored images to sell everything from toothpaste to political candidates. If one thinks the eccentric buffoon, for example, has no impact on the public, think of the backhanded compliment that so many psychiatrists hear from time to time: "You don't act like a psychiatrist." This comment is usually meant to imply that one behaves in a more or less normal, rational manner. Clearly, the underlying message is that the psychiatrist under consideration does not fit the cinematic stereotype of a neurotic, pompous, jargon-spouting weirdo.

If, as we are suggesting, the average person may not be adept at distinguishing the true nature of a particular occupation from its distorted image in the media, emotionally disturbed individuals will certainly have even greater difficulty. We have seen numerous clinical examples of this phenomenon. After viewing *One Flew Over the Cuckoo's Nest*, a patient in a psychiatric hospital revoked his previously given consent for electroconvulsive treatments. His psychiatrist explained, in vain, that the barbaric depiction in the movie was in no way similar to the modern version. Another patient, a female in analysis with a male analyst, saw the movie *Lovesick*, in which an analyst becomes sexually involved with his patient. After viewing the movie, she told her analyst that she was much more reluctant to talk about any erotic feelings that she might have toward her analyst. The movie made her feel that the professional boundaries between analyst and patient were much more permeable than she had thought.

A male patient seeing a female therapist might well assume that most female therapists are unfulfilled women more interested in finding a lover than a patient. Indeed, such was the case with a young professional man hospitalized for depression by a female psychiatrist. In the first few days of his hospitalization, he said to his psychiatrist, "I saw a movie where a woman doctor kissed her therapy patient to make him feel loved. I think it might help me if you would do that to me."

There is little doubt that the unempathic cold fish is a firmly entrenched stereotype in the minds of potential patients. After 1 month of psychotherapy, one patient told his therapist, "You must be different from most therapists. You react to what I say, you talk, you show emotion, you act human. I thought you would be 'the great stone face.' "

The stereotype of the repressive agent of society, for example, prevented one creative but severely disturbed artist from seeking treatment. He was convinced that any psychotherapist would demand that he give up his creativity in the service of adjusting and conforming to society's view of "well-adjusted behavior," a notion expressed most recently in Clint Eastwood's film about Charlie Parker, *Bird* (1989). The stereotype of the evil mind doctor may confirm some patients' view that psychiatrists really do not have their patients' best interests in mind. A frequent fantasy of paranoid patients is that they are being used for purposes of an unethical experiment without being told about it. A large number of movies would validate that this is a realistic concern when one seeks out a mental health professional. Similarly, a frequent transference fantasy in many, if not most, patients is that speaking in anger to their therapists will lead to retaliation. Hence the vindictive psychiatrist is repeatedly brought to life, if only in the fantasies of patients.

Even the rationalist foil depiction affects how patients may view their psychiatrists. This stereotype conveys an image of a cold, hyperrational scientist who is out of touch with the heart of man—that is, with the mysterious, spiritual transcendent dimension of the human psyche.

Just as negatively tinged stereotypes may lead patients to expect that their psychiatrists will somehow violate them, more positive portrayals may similarly result in patients developing unrealistic expectations of an idealized sort. For example, a young female college student who had seen *Ordinary People* came to therapy for a variety of problems in her relationships. After several weeks of therapy, she was growing increasingly irritated with her therapist. She insisted that he should behave more like Judd Hirsch in *Ordinary People*. Specifically, she wanted him to be less formal and hug her, as Judd Hirsch had embraced Timothy Hutton in the movie. The therapist explained his reasons for thinking that hugging her would not be in her best interest. She found his explanation unsatisfying and demanded, "If Judd Hirsch can do it, why can't you?" Her therapist maintained his position, and a split transference developed early in the psychotherapy, with the movie psychiatrist representing the idealized, all-good therapist, while the actual therapist was devalued as all bad.

Patients who have seen the blinding flash of insight from the cinematic version of the cathartic cure often expect similar results from their own psychotherapy. Numerous patients come to treatment fully expecting to engage in detective work, collaborating with their therapist to uncover the buried, traumatic memory that has created all their symptoms. These patients may ask to be hypnotized to facilitate the search for the missing link between etiology and cure. The belief that de-repressing a deep-seated, forgotten memory will lead to a cure can serve as a formidable resistance to therapeutic progress if patients repeatedly take flight from the here-and-now clinical situation in search of dark secrets from the past. Many patients express disappointment that after almost completing their treatments, they still have not experienced the catharsis so common in the movies.

If our culture's understanding of psychiatrists were derived entirely from the movies, the voluntary psychiatric patient would long ago have become extinct. The fact that the species is still extant may indicate that most Americans base their knowledge of the profession on a wider variety of sources. On the one hand, the enchanted medical mantle worn by psychiatrists may be largely impervious to assaults from the popular media. On the other hand, it is likely that the stigmatizing image of psychiatry in theatrical films is offset by the more positive, reassuring impression of psychotherapy that regularly appears on American television. Effective, appealingly human therapists have thrived in this medium, especially after the popular and critical success of *Ordinary People* in 1980. Even in the late 1960s, when the cinema was most critical of psychiatry, highly idealized therapists appeared in two weekly TV series, "Matt Lincoln" and "The Psychiatrist." More recently, Bob Newhart starred in a series about a therapist whose fallible but humane approach to therapy surely eased the anxieties of many a potential patient. We should also mention the long-running series "M*A*S*H," with its intrepid Dr. Sidney Freedman (played by Alan Arbus) as well as the innumerable made-for-TV films that produce competent therapists to solve problems associated with alcoholism, incest, teenage rebellion, bulimia, and the entire litany of troubling issues in American culture. In addition, television is populated with a variety of real-life therapists, many of whom are more dependent upon media appearances and book sales than on clinical practice. These therapists offer common sense advice to the large audiences for daytime and late-night talk shows. The typical American who is contemplating psychiatric treatment may willfully conjure up these televised images rather than the malevolent practitioners presented in *Cuckoo's Nest, Dressed to Kill,* and comparable films.

Nevertheless, psychiatry's image problems appear to have had a substantial effect on the young person contemplating a career in psychiatry. In fact, statistics reflecting patterns of medical student recruitment into the specialty of psychiatry parallel with uncanny synchrony the history of cinematic portrayals of psychiatrists that we have outlined (Gabbard and

Gabbard 1987). Beginning in 1965, there was a clear reduction in the number of medical school graduates specializing in psychiatry. This decline continued throughout the 1970s, when a 50% decrease in the percentage of graduates entering psychiatry was recorded by 1979. Yager and Scheiber (1981) found that the negative public image of psychiatry was a key factor in the decision of many students to avoid psychiatry as a specialty. They noted that media images of evil or foolish psychiatrists contributed to these negative feelings.

Federal funding of psychiatric research and education declined during the same time period in precisely the same historical pattern. Adjusting for inflation, National Institute of Mental Health grant support leveled off around the mid-1960s after almost two decades of significant increases (Pardes and Pincus 1983). This plateau was followed by a steady downturn from the mid-1960s to 1980.

The same pattern of decline and fall of the cinematic psychiatrist took place from the post–Golden Age year of 1964 to 1980, when there were almost consistently negative depictions of psychiatrists in movies. Whether the fall from grace in film is the partial cause or the partial result of these parallel patterns is a "chicken-egg" question that is probably unanswerable (Gabbard and Gabbard 1987). Presumably both processes mutually influence each other. While the movies cannot be entirely responsible for the prejudicial attitudes toward psychiatrists, they play a prominent role in perpetuating and broadening the stigma (Linter 1979).

Before concluding our discussion, we should note that psychiatric patients in American films have not fared any better than their treaters. The libidinous lecher stereotype has its counterpart in sex-starved, hysterical female patients depicted in films such as *Lilith* (1964) and *Spellbound* (1945). The evil mind doctor and the vengeful psychiatrist are mirrored in countless depictions of "homicidal maniacs" in slasher movies such as *Halloween* (1978). A handful of "mental patient" stereotypes seems to meet the needs of Hollywood storytellers so that the true complexity of mental illness rarely graces the screen.

Conclusion

We must recognize that the public at large has always maintained an ambivalent view of psychiatrists. On the one hand, there is awe at psychiatrists' understanding of the mysterious workings of the unconscious mind. Alongside this idealization and reverence, however, are contempt for their limitations, disappointment related to their inability to solve all the social ills of the world, and anger associated with their occasional failure even to solve the personal ills of the individual. Their perceived omniscience is envied and feared, so psychiatrists must be continually ridiculed and put down to neutralize these negative feelings. Movies reflect this process by seeking to demonstrate that psychiatrists are vulnerable to the same human frailties as everyone else. Psychiatrists may simply respond with, "So what? We already knew that." However, the fantasy that physicians specializing in psychiatry are somehow perfect or superior to everyone else dies hard. One is reminded of the humorous definition, "A psychoanalyst is someone who pretends he doesn't know everything" (Gabbard and Gabbard 1987, p. 172).

The choice of a career in psychiatry entails the acceptance that one must serve as a target for a variety of primitive feelings in one's patients. If therapists can accept that their roles as transference objects transcend the confines of the consulting room and spread onto the great silver screen, they can view the distortions with detached curiosity, with empathy, and with understanding, just as they approach transference attitudes in patients. In the meantime, psychiatrists can content themselves with the fact that the rash of films made about them reflects an intense interest in what we do on the part of filmmakers and on the part of film audiences. As we have noted previously in a paraphrase of Oscar Wilde, "The only thing worse than being portrayed in movies negatively is not being portrayed in movies at all" (Gabbard and Gabbard 1987, p. 173).

References

Fink PJ: The enigma of stigma and its relation to psychiatric education. Psychiatric Annals 13:669–690, 1983

Gabbard GO (ed): Sexual Exploitation in Professional Relationships. Washington, DC, American Psychiatric Press, 1989

Gabbard GO, Gabbard K: The female psychoanalyst in the movies. J Am Psychoanal Assoc 37:1031–1049, 1989

Gabbard K, Gabbard GO: Psychiatry and the Cinema. Chicago, IL, University of Chicago Press, 1987

Linter J: Reflections on the media and the mental patient. Hosp Community Psychiatry 30:415–416, 1979

Pardes H, Pincus H: Challenges to academic psychiatry. Psychiatry 140:1117–1126, 1983

Schneider I: Images of the mind: psychiatry in the commercial film. Am J Psychiatry 134:613–620, 1977

Schneider I: The theory and practice of movie psychiatry. Am J Psychiatry 144:996–1002, 1987

Yager J, Scheiber S: Why psychiatry is recruiting fewer residents: the opinions of medical school deans and psychiatric department chairmen. Journal of Psychiatric Education 5:258–268, 1981

Chapter 12

The Stigmatized Family

Harriet P. Lefley, Ph.D.

In this chapter the author identifies major sources of societal stigmatization of families of mentally ill persons and investigates the feelings of guilt, shame, embarrassment, confusion, anger, and fear that are consequences of stigma. Dr. Lefley points out that mental health professionals often intensify stigmatization by focusing on pathogenic rather than salutary elements in the family environment. Too often family therapists blame the family for the patient's illness. Thus, the suffering family is further burdened by the weight of blame.

Awareness of family issues has created new treatment efforts. Many mental health professionals have begun to promote a view of the family as ally and oppose interferences of dysfunctional family systems. Research findings, as well as the influence of the National Alliance for the Mentally Ill and its affiliates, are helping to change families' self concepts. Research has indicated that a sense of mastery is the single most important variable in alleviating family burdens. Families are now encouraged to become involved in support groups, planning, and advocacy, all of which contribute to destigmatization.

Stigmatization of mentally ill persons is a well-recognized cultural phenomenon that diminishes its victims, reinforces feelings of self-devaluation and alienation, and thus may well exacerbate or prolong the course of illness (Harding et al. 1987). Generalization of stigma to families is an additional source of psychological risk for both patients and their family members. Social barriers are frequently erected against the relatives and households of culturally devalued persons ranging from criminals to persons suffering from AIDS. In the case of mental illness, there are specific types of barriers that may affect the coping capacities of the patients' relatives and the staying powers of a needed support system. In his foreword to the book *Hidden Victims*, which deals with the reactions and healing process of families of the mentally ill, E. F. Torrey gives a potent description of some of these external pressures:

> Imagine what it would be like to have a member of your family afflicted with a condition whose sufferers, whenever the condition is depicted on television, are portrayed as violent 73 percent of the time, and homicidal 23 percent of the time. Imagine what it would be like to have your neighbors afraid to come to your house, and your children ashamed to bring their closest friends home to visit. Imagine having your relatives obliquely talking about your ill family member, unmistakably implying that your side of the family is guilty of something akin to original sin. No wonder Eugene O'Neill in *Strange Interlude* had the family hide their mentally ill aunt in the attic so that the family will not be disgraced. (Torrey 1988, pp. xi–xii)

Torrey's description embodies three major sources of societal stigmatization of families. The first, based on generalized fears of persons with mental illnesses, views the family home as a threatening place inhabited by a person with potentially harmful or highly offensive characteristics. The second source of stigma derives from blaming the family members and deeming them responsible for the patient's illness. And finally, there is shame by association, in which the family unit is viewed by the general public as an extension of the patient's deviance.

These aspects of stigma become part of the objective and subjective family burden. Objective burden refers to the external illness-related events that create hardships for families, and subjective burden refers to the degree of emotional distress elicited by these events (Noh and Turner 1987). Objective burdens of stigma may range from the community holding the family accountable for not being able to control the patient's aberrant behaviors, to condemnation and social ostracism of individual family members. Children with a mentally ill parent or sibling may be teased, maligned, and rejected by their peers. In many cases, mental illness in the family jeopardizes relationships with friends and neighbors; in extreme situations it may lead to almost total social isolation of the family unit (Dearth et al. 1986; Group for the Advancement of Psychiatry 1986; Lanquetot 1984; Rice et al. 1971).

Subjective burden—the family's distress over the pain and altered life prospects of their mentally ill relative—is exacerbated by these stigmatizing events. Reactions to perceived social censure become intertwined with responses to the sorrows and demands of the illness itself. Emotional reactions to major mental illness in a family member frequently include bewilderment, fear, denial, self-blame, sorrow, grieving, and empathic suffering (Lefley 1987c). The added perception of stigma may elicit rage and resentment or intensify depression and social withdrawal. Normative ambivalence toward mentally ill loved ones—the typical swing between exasperation provoked by the patient's behavior, guilt at the reaction, and sorrow evoked by the patient's suffering (Dearth et al. 1986; Group for the

Advancement of Psychiatry 1986)—may be exacerbated by social stigmatization of families. Thus, displaced anger because of the family's stress may coexist with identification with the patient's pain. And adding to the ambivalence in many cases is the intrapunitive internalization of societal beliefs about the family's role in mental illness.

Family Stigma

Internalized Stigma

Guilt is the most prevalent manifestation of internalized stigma. There is evidence of irrational parental guilt across a range of disabilities, from mental retardation (Turnbull and Turnbull 1978) to cerebral palsy (McCubbin et al. 1982). In mental illness, however, parents have learned of "crazymaking families" through the media, often reinforced by clear messages of their own culpability from the experts who treat their loved ones (Francell et al. 1988; Group for the Advancement of Psychiatry 1986; Lefley 1989). Certainly there is no greater self-stigmatization than the conviction that, however inadvertently, one has caused a devastating, life-diminishing illness in a loved one. In a study of stigma among 487 members of the National Alliance for the Mentally Ill (NAMI), about one-fifth of the respondents, primarily mothers, reported that their self-esteem had been much or very much damaged by stigma. This stigma was attributed to public beliefs about parental roles in causing the disorder. In a similar number of cases, stigma resulted in disrupted family relationships with other family members as well as with the mentally ill relatives (Wahl and Harman 1989).

Even among those who have finally decided they did not cause the illness (Hatfield 1981), there is residual guilt for failure to recognize symptoms or to seek help early enough, for being too easily provoked, for having expectations that seemed age-appropriate but perhaps were too demanding, or generally for lacking the foresight that might have prevented an unimaginable decompensation—regardless of whether it occurred at home, at school, or in another city far away (Lefley 1987c).

With chronic patients there are ongoing sources of guilt based on family members' need to establish limits on self-sacrifice. Families feel guilty about involuntary commitment of loved ones whose behavior may be life-threatening; for calling the police despite great provocation or need; for placing relatives in hospitals or in community residences that are inferior to their own homes; for withholding money that the patient is likely to lose or squander; or simply for trying to live their own lives free of turmoil and pain (Lefley 1987a, 1987c). In almost all situations requiring self-protective decisions, families must deal with the patient's resentment and with their own ambivalence about depriving a loved one whose life is impoverished compared with their own. Many people tend to feel like "bad parents" or "bad siblings" when they must make these difficult choices.

There are other types of internalized stigma. Some families of persons with severe disabilities, including those who are psychiatrically disabled, feel they have been selected for misfortune because of some unknown taint or ancestral crime. A few persons have verbalized this feeling in support groups of families of mentally ill persons. Equally destructive is the self-stigmatization of the "bad seed." In families with a history of serious mental illness, some members feel that their lineage has been "cursed" by malevolent fate despite an overt knowledge of genetic vulnerability and the randomness of disease distributions in family pedigrees. For others, misinformed views of the genetic odds may generate a conviction that they have a high potential for decompensation. Some siblings and adult children exaggerate their own vulnerability and are overattentive to imaginary prodromal cues. There are fears for oneself and for one's future children, affecting marital and reproductive decisions. In a few fearful parents, there is stigmatic projection of the family curse and hypervigilance toward symptoms in unaffected children and grandchildren.

Children's Feelings of Stigmatization

There is evidence from research and from first-person accounts in the literature that children and adolescents frequently feel stigmatized because of the mental illness of a parent or sibling. A comprehensive study of 652 children from 253 families with a seriously mentally ill parent found that the following variables affected children's feelings about themselves: chaotic households, verbal and physical abuse, children's need to restrain parents to prevent harm to the parent or themselves or to protect property, and shame and embarrassment. There were also two varieties of identification with the aggressor. One phenomenon involved children joining peers to laugh at the bizarre behavior of their own mentally ill parent—allying with the stigmatizers rather than with the stigmatized. The other phenomenon involved symptom modeling, mimicking the paranoid or self-destructive behavior of the mentally ill parent (Rice et al. 1971).

First-person accounts of children of psychotic parents indicate memories of shame, embarrassment, confusion, anger, fear, and even terror. Frequently reported are memories of a lack of trust because of the parent's inability to maintain consistent control of cognition or affect. These negative feelings often alternated with positive memories of love and kindness, making it difficult to integrate good and bad introjects and perhaps establishing the groundwork for splitting in a vulnerable child. Feelings of "badness," both because of the parent's tirades against the child and the child's fear of being like the parent, are often reported (Lanquetot 1984).

Among siblings, fears, shame, and feelings of loss are common phenomena. There are fears of coinheritance or of being "different" like the ill sibling, and fears of inheriting the problem after the parents are gone (Moorman 1988). Shame and feelings of stigmatization are evoked by the aversive behaviors of the mentally ill family member. Siblings report objective problems of loss of friends, popularity, and reputation. Among many, there is mourning for a well-loved premorbid personality that is now but a dim memory. There are feelings of deprivation and loss both of the brother or sister they knew and of the person he or she might have become—the experience of dual loss (Lefley 1987c). Guilt is almost always reported by the well siblings: for the divergent developmental paths and the relative richness of their lives compared with the impoverished fortunes of siblings who once were close; for not doing more to alleviate the burden on parental caregivers; and for the distancing that typically becomes a major adaptive strategy as they try to fulfill their own destinies (Brodoff 1988; Group for the Advancement of Psychiatry 1986; Moorman 1988).

Unfortunately, unless the relatives present themselves for therapy to process the impact of the patient's illness, mental health professionals have little awareness of these pressures on families. Significant sources of family stigma include etiological theories that have trickled down through the popular media, exclusionary policies of the provider system, and the negative views of families still found among many practitioners.

Stigmatization by Professionals

Increasing numbers of clinicians, psychiatrists in particular, have expressed their chagrin over the mistreatment of families by mental health professionals (Appleton 1974; Grunebaum 1986; Lamb 1983). Many families have reported their anger, despair, and feelings of stigmatization after interactions with clinicians ranging from studied evasion to outright hostility (Dearth et al. 1986; Group for the Advancement of Psychiatry 1986; Lefley 1989; Walsh 1985). Goldstein (1981) has described the message sometimes conveyed to families: that "the patient's illness was their fault and they should go away, shrouded in guilt, and leave the professional to undo the damage" (p. 2).

Proliferation of biogenetic research findings and an emerging literature on the parameters of family burden have somewhat softened the older prejudices against families, but the concept of parental toxicity still has wide currency in the field. The concept of the "schizophrenogenic mother" has largely been disavowed. Arieti (1981) claimed that in his long years of practice with schizophrenic patients, only 20% to 25% of the mothers he saw bore any resemblance to that description. Yet in grand rounds and case presentations we continue to hear the term "schizophrenogenic mother" used to describe the behavior of a particular kind of woman, sometimes accompanied by the laughing demur, "Of course I don't believe that mothers cause schizophrenia!"

In contrast to other areas of learning or of medicine, in mental health practice some internal connection is invariably drawn between observed behaviors of family members and the patient's condition. And the inference is almost automatically unidirectional and causal—family to patient— rather than correlational or reactive. Despite the failure of a quarter-century of research to demonstrate familial etiology of the major psychoses (Howells and Guirguis 1985), most of us have been trained to analyze the family's behavior as contributing to the patient's symptomatology, highlighting negative behaviors and ignoring positive interactions.

As Arieti (1981) has suggested, many therapists have taken at face value and reinforced their schizophrenic patients' negative descriptions of their parents without questioning why favorable memories have been ignored or withheld. Terkelsen (1983) has noted that despite their systemic view, many family therapists cannot function without an implicit explanatory model that blames the family for the illness. "Blame," Terkelsen points out, "is avoided only at the expense of conceptual clarity—by declining to address the issue of etiology altogether" (p. 194).

In the main, diagnostic assessments and case reports tend to focus on pathogenic rather than on salutary elements in the patients' environments. Consider the research on expressed emotion (EE) and the emphasis on the criticalness and emotional overinvolvement of families with high EE, rather than the calm, benign affects of families with low EE—despite the fact that low EE is far more prevalent in most studies of families of persons with schizophrenia (Jenkins et al. 1986; Leff and Vaughn 1985). Moreover, the investigators of EE explicitly have disavowed any inferences of family causation in schizophrenia and have emphasized the need for research in nonfamilial environments (Vaughn et al. 1984).

Family members who experience a psychotic episode in a loved one are typically suffering great pain and bewilderment. When they are excluded from the information and treatment process and given a negative message of their own role, and when this process recurs over many years of illness, defensive strategies may develop in dealing with service providers. These may include anticipatory, aggressive, or demanding behaviors because of learned expectations of evasiveness or rejection. Relatives who have lived through years of treatment and financial impoverishment, without perceived benefit, may displace their cumulative frustrations onto each new psychiatric resident who rediagnoses the patient for the "nth" time. Alternatively, some mothers may act overly humble or passive to avoid being stereotyped as intrusive or controlling.

In the complex psychodynamics of family-clinician interactions, some family members may actually seek to fulfill perceived negative expectancies of clinicians (Lefley 1989). The reasons given are fascinating and often insightful. In anecdotal reports of their reactions during crisis interventions, relatives have recalled displaying aversive behaviors that they realized were aimed at confirming the clinician's bias but were actually atypical and ego-alien. "She seemed to assume that I was an interfering mother and I found myself meeting her needs," a usually mild woman recalled about her interaction with a social worker. "I started asking her all kinds of questions about treatment even though I knew the answers already." A burnt-out sibling confessed that she deliberately acted hostile so that the crisis-admissions resident might then feel sorry for the patient and admit her to one of the few beds on the inpatient unit. On a more complex level, one insightful parent theorized about his own psychodynamics in unexpectedly acting like a domineering father, which he saw as an ego-dystonic role: "One, I may actually be a domineering father underneath; or two, I want to believe I can control this terrible situation. But my acting up also provides a rationale for my son's illness in the psychiatrist's eyes. So now maybe he [the psychiatrist] can help him."

Some parents felt that aversive behavior would corroborate their own guilty role in precipitating the crisis: "If I was the bad one, then I could change my behavior and Arthur would get well." Terkelsen (1982) has described this as "the magical aspect of the wish to be blamed" (p. 183). He has similarly described working with parents who cling to theories of family pathogenesis because this explanatory model provides a means of expiation and approval by authority figures with the power of healing their child.

Psychodynamic issues that plague the family-clinician relationship were even evident in a study of 84 seasoned mental health professionals with seriously mentally ill relatives (Lefley 1987d). In this study only 26% of the sample were willing to talk openly about the illness with colleagues; 48% were guarded; and 26% expressed strong reluctance. More than 90% of the respondents indicated that they frequently heard colleagues make disparaging remarks about patients' families; yet almost one-third admitted that although they disagreed, they remained silent. The majority were ambivalent about any participant role in the case, even when they felt they had information or expertise that might contribute to successful outcome. Most questioned theories of family pathogenesis, siblings even more than parents, and many expressed anger at the insensitivity of practitioners to families' pain (Lefley 1985a). Overall, role conflict appeared to be associated with perceived stigma from colleagues.

Cross-Cultural Aspects of Family Stigma

The cross-cultural literature indicates that stigmatization of mentally ill persons and their families is less pronounced in traditional cultures (Lefley 1985b, 1987b). True, there is a history of isolation and even of abandonment of persons with severe, prolonged illnesses in some nonwestern cultures, and many families feel shamed by the aberrant behaviors of one of their members. Nevertheless, a number of cross-cultural observers have proposed that stigma is less prevalent in cultures that attribute psychiatric symptoms to somatic or supernatural causes (Lin and Kleinman 1988) or even, in some contexts, endow these symptoms with positive religious value. This view tends to free both patient and family of blame, generating less social rejection and self-devaluation of patients.

In contrast to western etiological theories and exclusionary policies, it is evident from the world psychiatric literature that families are considered valued allies in most traditional cultures (Bell 1982; DiNicola 1985; Lefley 1985b, 1987b). In fact, it would be incongruent not to involve the family in diagnostic information and treatment decisions regarding the patient. Johnson (1989) has described the salutary influence of biogenic findings on the self concept of families of mentally ill persons in our own culture. In the nonwestern world view, externalized causality and somatic/supernatural explanations similarly free families of stigma. In addition, values of interdependence and extended kinship structure, and professionals' willingness to work collaboratively with families, are viewed as some of the cultural strengths that may mediate the course of illness (Lefley 1990; Lin and Kleinman 1988).

Reducing Family Stigma

Professional Training

Despite a great deal of enlightenment, clinical training programs continue to assign contemporary texts that incorporate notions of family etiology and "schizophrenogenic" parents as viable causal hypotheses in the major psychoses (e.g., Carson et al. 1988). Systems-oriented theories that assign a functional value to schizophrenic symptomatology for family homeostasis are also widely taught. Family therapy has not had notable success in the case of schizophrenia and has largely abandoned the population with which it began. Nevertheless, new generations of clinicians continue to learn inappropriate techniques for working with chronic patients, and these teachings provide an ongoing rationale for projecting frustrations and ascribing lack of progress to family resistance and sabotage.

There are, however, salutary trends in professional training that are teaching new skills and techniques in working with families and are promoting a view of families as allies in the treatment process (Lefley and Johnson 1990). Psychoeducational interventions, despite their continuing emphasis on the relationship of familial behavior to decompensation, nevertheless have shifted the approach from systemic manipulation to meeting families' expressed needs for information, support, behavior management, and problem-solving techniques. Moreover, psychoeducators seem actively opposed to inferences of dysfunctional family systems and presumptive psychopathology (Anderson et al. 1986; Falloon et al. 1984; Goldstein 1981). Some of us have proposed a model of stress, coping, and adaptation in working with families. Here the emphasis is on education, support, and advocacy so that families can not only deal with the illnesses but also become actively involved in changing the external conditions that affect their lives (Hatfield and Lefley 1987).

A number of National Institute of Mental Health (NIMH) national conferences have been held to promote training of clinicians for work with seriously mentally ill patients and their families (Lefley et al. 1989). A tri-state multidisciplinary training grant is specifically oriented toward training clinicians in three core professions—psychiatry, psychology, and social work—to work in a collaborative model with families of seriously mentally ill persons (Lefley 1988). Collaborative approaches in family therapy have been proposed (Terkelsen 1982, 1983), including a model of systems consultation that is specifically tuned to families' formulation of needs (Wynne et al. 1986). Family members are also training mental health professionals by sharing their experiences and expertise in preservice graduate courses and in continuing education. Members of the NAMI Curriculum and Training Network have had invited roles as lecturers, grand rounds discussants, workshop conductors, and presenters at national and state conferences. The NIMH, through its clinical training and community support systems grants, has regularly required consumer and family input, in areas ranging from faculty and curriculum development to models of service delivery.

Changing Families' Self Concept

New biogenetic research findings that have found their way into the popular media have affected the way families view themselves and their role in mental illness (Johnson 1989). The remarkable growth and influence of NAMI and its affiliates have also had a pronounced effect, both directly and indirectly, on families' perception of stigma in their loved ones and in themselves. Increasingly, respected clinicians are absolving families of blame (Lamb 1983) and calling for collaborative alliances with families (Grunebaum 1986). Cultural views of mentally ill persons are changing with increasing media exposure of genetic and brain research, and programs that feature families or recovered patients. Families who participate in support groups are learning to ventilate and absolve themselves of old guilts and fears. Sharing experiences with others reduces self-blaming and feelings of culpability. Group members also teach one another new techniques for dealing with difficult situations, convey resource information, empathize with one another's pain, and mutually shore up their adaptive strengths.

Many regulatory agencies are now mandating involvement of families in treatment and discharge planning. Family members are solicited to become members of advisory and governance boards of mental health agencies, to do monitoring and evaluation, and to participate in mental health systems planning and grant reviews at state and federal levels. Participation in the planning process and advocacy for research, resources, and services tend to diminish the former sense of helplessness and despair. Research has indicated that a sense of mastery is the single most important variable in alleviating family burden (Noh and Turner 1987). Planning and advocacy are important mechanisms for improving family members' self concept and for enhancing their control of the events that shape their lives and those of their loved ones.

All of these efforts contribute to destigmatization. Public involvement and proud advocacy for the needs and rights of mentally ill persons are actions that affect social stigma and attenuate its personal impact. Self-stigmatization diminishes as family members begin to appreciate their own levels of knowledge and efficacy. In many cases, as mental health professionals and family members increasingly meet and function on a collaborative basis, clinicians' views of families are changing from assumptions of pathogenesis to admiration for the families' dedication, breadth of information, and coping strengths under conditions of great adversity.

References

Anderson C, Reiss D, Hogarty G: Schizophrenia and the Family: A Practitioner's Guide to Psychoeducation and Management. New York, Guilford, 1986

Appleton WS: Mistreatment of patients' families by psychiatrists. Am J Psychiatry 131:655–657, 1974

Arieti S: The family of the schizophrenic and its participation in the therapeutic task, in American Handbook of Psychiatry, 2nd Edition, Vol 7. Edited by Arieti S, Brodie KH. New York, Basic Books, 1981, pp 271–284

Bell J: The family in the hospital: experiences in other countries, in The Psychiatric Hospital and the Family. Edited by Harbin H. New York, Spectrum, 1982, pp 255–276

Brodoff AS: First person account: schizophrenia through a sister's eyes—the burden of invisible baggage. Schizophr Bull 14:113–116, 1988

Carson RC, Butcher JN, Coleman JC: Abnormal Psychology and Modern Life, 8th Edition. Glenview, IL, Scott Foresman, 1988

Dearth N, Labenski BJ, Mott ME, et al: Families Helping Families: Living With Schizophrenia. New York, WW Norton, 1986

DiNicola VF: Family therapy and transcultural psychiatry: an emerging synthesis, Part I: The conceptual basis. Transcultural Psychiatric Research Review 22:81–113, 1985

Falloon IRH, Boyd JL, McGill CW: Family Care of Schizophrenia. New York, Guilford, 1984

Francell CG, Conn VS, Gray DP: Families' perceptions of burden of care for chronic mentally ill relatives. Hosp Community Psychiatry 39:1296–1300, 1988

Goldstein MJ (ed): New Developments in Interventions With Families of Schizophrenics. New Directions in Mental Health Services, No 12. San Francisco, CA, Jossey-Bass, 1981

Group for the Advancement of Psychiatry: A Family Affair: Helping Families Cope With Mental Illness—A Guide for the Professions. Report No 119. New York, Brunner/Mazel, 1986

Grunebaum H: Families, patients, and mental health professionals: toward a new collaboration. Am J Psychiatry 143:1420–1421, 1986

Harding CM, Zubin J, Strauss JS: Chronicity in schizophrenia: fact, partial fact, or artifact? Hosp Community Psychiatry 38:477–486, 1987

Hatfield AB: Coping effectiveness in families of the mentally ill: an exploratory study. Journal of Psychiatric Treatment and Evaluation 3:11–19, 1981

Hatfield AB, Lefley HP (eds): Families of the Mentally Ill: Coping and Adaptation. New York, Guilford, 1987

Howells JF, Guirguis WR: The Family and Schizophrenia. Madison, CT, International Universities Press, 1985

Jenkins JH, Karno M, de la Selva A, et al: Expressed emotion in cross-cultural context: familial responses to schizophrenia among Mexican Americans, in Treatment of Schizophrenia: Family Assessment and Intervention. Edited by Goldstein MJ. Berlin, Springer-Verlag, 1986, pp 35–49

Johnson DL: Schizophrenia as a brain disease: implications for psychologists and families. Am Psychol 44:553–555, 1989

Lamb HR: Families: practical help replaces blame. Hosp Community Psychiatry 34:893, 1983

Lanquetot R: First-person account: confessions of the daughter of a schizophrenic. Schizophr Bull 10:467–471, 1984

Leff J, Vaughn C: Expressed Emotion in Families. New York, Guilford, 1985

Lefley HP: Etiological and prevention views of clinicians with mentally ill relatives. Am J Orthopsychiatry 55:363–370, 1985a

Lefley HP: Families of the mentally ill in cross-cultural perspective. Psychosocial Rehabilitation Journal 8:57–75, 1985b

Lefley HP: Aging parents as caregivers of mentally ill adult children: an emerging social problem. Hosp Community Psychiatry 38:1063–1070, 1987a

Lefley HP: Culture and mental illness: the family role, in Families of the Mentally Ill: Coping and Adaptation. Edited by Hatfield AB, Lefley HP. New York, Guilford, 1987b, pp 30–59

Lefley HP: The family's response to mental illness in a relative, in Families of the Mentally Ill: Meeting the Challenges. New Directions in Mental Health Services, No 34. San Francisco, Jossey-Bass, 1987c, pp 3–21

Lefley HP: Impact of mental illness in families of mental health professionals. J Nerv Ment Dis 175:613–619, 1987d

Lefley HP: Training mental health professionals to work with families of chronic patients. Community Ment Health J 24:338–357, 1988

Lefley HP: Family burden and family stigma in major mental illness. Am Psychol 44:556–560, 1989

Lefley HP: Culture and chronic mental illness. Hosp Community Psychiatry 41:277–286, 1990

Lefley HP, Johnson DL: Families as Allies in Treatment of the Mentally Ill: New Directions for Mental Health Professionals. Washington DC, American Psychiatric Press, 1990

Lefley HP, Bernheim KF, Goldman CR: National forum addresses need to enhance training in treating the seriously mentally ill. Hosp Community Psychiatry 40:460–462, 470, 1989

Lin K-M, Kleinman AM: Psychopathology and clinical course of schizophrenia: a cross-cultural perspective. Schizophr Bull 14:555–567, 1988

McCubbin HI, Nevin RS, Cauble AE, et al: Family coping with chronic illness: the case of cerebral palsy, in Family Stress, Coping, and Social Support. Edited by McCubbin HI, Cauble AE, Patterson JM. Springfield, IL, Charles C Thomas, 1982, pp 169–188

Moorman M: A sister's need. New York Times Magazine, Sept 11, 1988, pp 44–46, 50–53, 116

Noh S, Turner RJ: Living with psychiatric patients: implications for the mental health of family members. Soc Sci Med 25:263–271, 1987

Rice EP, Ekdahl MC, Miller L: Children of Mentally Ill Parents. New York, Behavorial Publications, 1971

Terkelsen KG: The straight approach to a knotty problem: managing parental guilt about psychosis, in Questions and Answers in the Practice of Family Therapy, Vol 2. Edited by Gurman AS. New York, Brunner/Mazel, 1982, pp 179–183

Terkelsen KG: Schizophrenia and the family, II: Adverse effects of family therapy. Fam Process 22:191–200, 1983

Torrey EF: Foreword, in Hidden Victims: An Eight-Stage Healing Process for Families and Friends of the Mentally Ill. New York, Doubleday, 1988, pp xi–xiii

Turnbull AP, Turnbull HR: Parents Speak Out: Views From the Other Side of the Two-Way Mirror. Columbus, OH, Charles E Merrill, 1978

Vaughn CE, Snyder KS, Jones S, et al: Family factors in schizophrenic relapse. Arch Gen Psychiatry 41:1169–1177, 1984

Wahl OW, Harman CR: Family views of stigma. Schizophr Bull 15:131–139, 1989

Walsh M: Schizophrenia: Straight Talk for Families and Friends. New York, Morrow, 1985

Wynne LC, McDaniel SH, Weber TT: Systems Consultation: A New Perspective for Family Therapy. New York, Guilford, 1986

Chapter 13

Fighting Stigma: How to Help the Doctor's Family

Michael F. Myers, M.D., F.R.C.P.(C)

In this chapter, Dr. Myers describes his clinical observations of psychiatrically ill doctors and their families struggling with mental illness.

Dr. Myers examines the issues of denial, shame, disruption of family homeostasis, and fear and avoidance of treatment, with a focus on issues that apply particularly to physicians and their families. His brief case histories dramatically highlight his observations. Dr. Myers recommends that the treating psychiatrist become more aware of the ignorance and naiveté about psychiatric illness in doctors and their families. Too often families are left uninformed because the psychiatrist assumes their understanding and knowledge.

Dr. Myers also recommends a family-systems approach to the understanding and treatment of these families. Such an approach uncovers the "shaming system" that operates as a form of behavioral control. The family-systems perspective facilitates treatment that includes spouses, parents, and children of disturbed patients. Dr. Myers concludes with an assertion that psychiatrists must be advocates for both the mentally ill patient and the entire family.

In this chapter I describe some of my clinical observations of psychiatrically ill doctors and their families. These observations are from a large sample of approximately 300 medical students and doctors whom I have assessed and treated over the past 15 years of psychiatric practice. They are a heterogenous group of doctors with a range of DSM-III-R (American Psychiatric Association 1987) diagnoses from the most benign to the most severely disabling. The gender mix is roughly one-third female and two-thirds male. The sample is largely heterosexual doctors who are single, married, or divorced, but there is a significant minority who are gay male or lesbian physicians, with or without life partners. Although I am reporting here exclusively on physicians and their families, many of my findings are generalizable to any individual with psychiatric illness and his or her family.

Denial of Illness

Denial of psychiatric illness is not uncommon in doctors, nor is it uncommon in doctors' families. In some marriages there may be a collusive denial in spouses that either or both have a psychiatric problem; in some families there may be a collective denial among all members that the physician family member is ill. Examples might include the alcoholic physician whose wife denies and protects him from possible censure by covering up for him (she may or may not have a drinking problem herself); the depressed woman physician who has insight into her illness but whose husband denies its existence or magnitude and may unconsciously undermine her efforts to seek proper care; and the depressed and suicidal medical student or resident whose parents deny that he or she is depressed.

Understanding the family dynamics can assist the clinician tremendously in treating the physician with a psychiatric illness. One must not underestimate the degree of anxiety (and the defenses against that anxiety) in the families of doctors as they grapple with stigmatization. This anxiety may be particularly manifested in those physician families who reside in rural communities, but it is also seen in families living in cities where the physician has a high profile professionally. Apart from these more sociocultural dynamics that color a doctor family's reaction to illness, many medical families operate with a family ethos of privacy, dignity, pride, and "normalcy" at all costs. In these families, there may be a very high drive for excellence and achievement in all family members. There may also be a host of family secrets that are not to be breached. Some families with lengthy and prominent medical lineage may have little tolerance of, or empathy for, a doctor-relative with a psychiatric illness.

Case Example 1

Dr. and Mrs. A. came to see me at the urging of their 23-year-old son who was called to the family home after Dr. A. had physically assaulted his wife. Dr. A. had driven home at 4 A.M. intoxicated after a late poker game with several other doctors. He awakened his wife after smashing into the garage door that he thought was open. Dr. A. struck his wife with his fist (resulting in a black eye) when Mrs. A. confronted him about drinking and driving. Although Dr. A. had at least a 10-year history of an established drinking problem with morning shakes, alcoholic blackouts, and one warning for impaired driving, he had never sought help. Likewise, Mrs. A. had never spoken to her family physician or gone to Alanon despite repeated exhortations from her four adult children.

Case Example 2

Dr. B., a pathologist, was referred to me by his family physician for confirmation of a mood disorder. He had been symptomatic for 4 months with terminal insomnia, morning dread, anhedonia, a 15-pound weight loss, lethargy, and guilt about leaning too heavily on his research associate to do so much of his work. A complete history and mental status exam rendered a diagnosis of depression. I started him on a tricyclic antidepressant with an appointment to return in 1 week. The following day he canceled his appointment through my secretary and gave no explanation. When I called him he told me that his wife, a general practitioner, was very upset when he told her that he had come to see me: "She said that I'm not depressed, that I don't need medication, and that I shouldn't be wasting a busy psychiatrist's precious time. She and I are going to do yoga together."

Case Example 3

Mr. C., a third-year medical student, came to see me for "psychotherapy and possibly medication." He began the first visit by addressing the matter of confidentiality in the doctor-patient relationship. More specifically, he had come to see me against the wishes of his father, a psychiatrist on the faculty of our medical school, and he wanted to be certain that I would not discuss his situation with his father. He had on several occasions asked his father about seeing a psychiatrist because of general unhappiness in his life and social inhibitions and isolation. His father downplayed his son's need to see someone and said that he was suffering from "normal medical student stress" and told him not to worry. At the end of our first session, Mr. C. asked if dysthymic disorders were hereditary. When I asked him about the question, he shamefully told me that he had inadvertently stumbled upon a bottle of phenelzine in his father's dresser drawer several months earlier when he was looking to borrow a sweater.

Ignorance and Naiveté in Doctors' Families

Sometimes ignorance and/or naiveté about psychiatric illness may be confused with denial. In some families, both may be present. I am referring here to situations in which the doctor's family really does lack information, or the family members are misinformed, or they have outdated information about psychiatric disorders and their treatment. Several examples come to mind: the role of genetics in alcoholism; the biological underpinnings of clinical depression; the indications for antidepressants and their differentiation from habit-forming drugs; and the various forms of psychotherapy. Sometimes the family has not realized that physicians are human, too, and are therefore subject to the whole gamut of illnesses.

The clinician must realize that it is not only nonmedical relatives of doctors who may lack information and understanding about psychiatric problems; many doctor-relatives have a similar lack of knowledge. These doctors may not do clinical work; they may instead be in a very different branch of medicine, or they may have done their undergraduate training in psychiatry many years earlier. Even when the spouse, parent, or adult child of a psychiatrically impaired physician is a psychiatrist himself or herself, that person may be in a psychiatric subspecialty or may practice a particular form of psychiatry that is quite different from the treatment of choice for the ill physician. I emphasize this because of the many occasions when I have consulted on cases in which the treating doctor erroneously assumed that medically trained relatives knew all about their loved one's illness and did not require any explanation and/or support. In those situations, the physician-patient's family often felt disgruntled with the treating physician, and he or she in turn was annoyed with and disbelieving of the family.

Shame

I have found that the more serious the diagnosis of psychiatric impairment, the greater the felt sense of stigmatization in the physician and his or her family. This is especially so in those doctors who are on medication (in whom the degree of subjective stigmatization may vary with the type of drug, the dosage, the length of time on the drug, and so forth), those who are on medical leave from their work, those who have been admitted to a psychiatric facility, and those who have entered a residential treatment setting for alcohol or other drug abuse. Many of these men and women feel ashamed and inadequate as physicians.

Just as doctors who struggle with their psychiatric problems experience shame, so do their relatives. Will (1987) has described shame as

> a painful, unpleasant emotion experienced as an accompaniment of some awareness of wrong-doing, impropriety, shortcoming, or transgression of behavior and concepts of what is held to be "right," "good," or acceptable within a particular group. It is equated with feelings of disgrace, dishonor, infamy, humiliation, odium, or the like, and may be accompanied by physical sensations of apprehension, disgust, nausea, and dread. To be ashamed is to be faced with censure and the possible removal of the human support that is felt as necessary to exist with some semblance of comfort. (p. 309)

Many of the clauses contained in this brief passage embody the intense feelings that some family members have when their physician-relative is ill. And herein lies the catch-22 for doctors. As long as doctors are revered as omnipotent, unsullied, and beyond reproach, it is impossible for them or their relatives not to feel a sense of shame when they become ill. The stigmatization is ubiquitous—in the doctors themselves, in their families, in the medical community, in the community at large, and even in us, the caregivers. If one takes a systems approach to the problem of shame in the psychiatrically impaired doctor, then one can see that the "shaming system" (in which shame is used as a form of behavioral control) is quite pronounced in many medical families and in the institution of medicine itself.

Case Example 1

Mrs. D., the wife of a medical specialist, came to see me for many symptoms suggestive of a panic disorder with agoraphobia. Although Mrs. D. described a long history of nervousness and worry, she had never before been this symptomatic. The precipitant to her illness was her husband's dismissal as a divisional head of an academic department at a local medical school. He had been dismissed because of several sexual harassment charges against him by female nurses and medical students. Mrs. D. felt a profound degree of shame in the context of the department in which her husband worked, in particular, with all of the spouses that she had known over the years. She also felt humiliated in the ethnic minority group in which she and her husband were very prominent.

Case Example 2

Dr. E. was a 48-year-old internist who suffered from a severe bipolar illness. During one quite protracted admission to our psychiatric unit, he requested an evening pass to attend his daughter's graduation exercises from high school. His daughter was the class valedictorian and he was excited to attend. Late in the afternoon, I received a phone call from Mrs. E. (from whom Dr. E. had recently separated) saying that her daughter was refusing to attend the graduation if her father was going to be there. She was embarrassed that her friends and teachers would notice that he looked "like a mental case." Indeed, her father was still quite depressed and visibly ill. He had a lot of psychomotor retardation, a staring gaze, and a movement disorder from his many psychotropic medications.

Case Example 3

Although Mr. F. initially came to see me for couple therapy with his wife, it quickly emerged that what he needed and wanted was individual therapy. Mr. F. had many unresolved issues stemming from his background, much anger about his parents' marriage (his parents were both physicians), and separation-individuation problems with his mother. After several weeks of therapy, Mr. F. announced that he had to start being more honest with me. What he meant by that was that his father was a wife-batterer and both Mr. F. and his mother engaged in a secret pact to never tell anyone because of their image as a medical family in a small community. To protect his mother, Mr. F. would frequently intercede as a boy and take beatings himself. Dr. F. would berate his son for "being a mommy's boy" and "a potential faggot." On a couple of occasions when Dr. F. was in a drunken rage, he forced his son to strip naked while he beat him and scoffed at him about the size of his penis. Mr. F. told me that because I was a doctor myself he feared that I wouldn't believe his story.

Disruption of Family Homeostasis

There can be monumental fallout in the doctor's family when he or she becomes psychiatrically ill. Loss of income occurs when the doctor is not able to practice medicine at all or to the degree that he or she practiced before becoming ill. Disability insurance helps, but there may be a lot of anxiety about expenses and changes in life-style for all members of the family. If a male physician is in a traditional marriage, his wife may have to return to paid work outside the home when she is not prepared for it either psychologically or occupationally. That is, if there is not work available for her in the field in which she trained several years earlier, she may have to accept unskilled work that pays poorly and may be humiliating for her. She may suffer reentry anxiety, and a disruption in the domestic equilibrium at home may result that will require a period of adjustment for all family members.

For married women doctors, the loss of income will require a period of budgetary adjustment even when their husbands have well-paying jobs or professions. For single-parent women doctors (and there are many of these), the financial headaches may become a nightmare, and this in turn may adversely affect their ability to heal from their illnesses. Their educational debt load coupled with child care expenses may be overwhelming. Many single-parent women doctors are living close to the economic edge; a large number of them are receiving no (or inadequate) child support payments from their ex-husbands. Because these women are members of a professional group, mythology abounds about their financial autonomy.

Another type of fallout for the family when the physician member becomes ill is psychological. Specifically, there may be a felt assault to one's perception of the physician spouse or parent as invulnerable and larger than life. The family must then enter a period of mourning for whatever the idealized image of the family was as they come to terms with what the future might hold in the sense of changed expectations of constancy.

It is well documented that people with psychiatric disorders are prone to marital conflict and divorce (Briscoe and Smith 1973). All psychiatrists have seen couples and families torn apart by the pervasive effects of some types of psychiatric illness. One of the most common situations that marital therapists see in their practices is an undiagnosed depression in one or both partners that neither has recognized. Instead of seeing the spouse as ill, the partner sees him or her as bad, lazy, or uncaring. It behooves the clinician who is looking after a physician with a primary psychiatric illness to keep an eye on the doctor's marriage as well. The family members will all be adjusting to a new life in some way, a life that may be quite different from that which they had before the illness or from what they had imagined the future would be. The physician may need to leave a prestigious position or a lucrative practice for a less stressful medical life-style. The family may have to relocate geographically. There may be many debts. There may be much anger and resentment among family members about so many changes. There may be many splits and alliances within the family, both the immediate and the extended family.

Case Example 1

Dr. G., a 36-year-old psychiatrist, came to see me for marital therapy with her 38-year-old attorney husband. In the course of my individual history-taking session with her, she told me about her fears of bipolar illness in herself since her father was a manic-depressive whose first episode occurred when he was in his forties. Ironically, she was a final-year medical student doing an elective in psychiatry when her father, a radiologist, went into an acute manic state.

Her mother called Dr. G. to come over because her father was acting very strangely. She recalled:

> I will never forget walking into our family home and seeing my mother in tears. My father was talking nonstop about absolutely nothing and laughing hilariously about something that made sense only to him. I remember doing some sort of mental status exam on him; then suddenly I slugged him. I don't know where the impulse came from. I wanted to knock him out of this crazy state and bring him back to us. And I remember screaming at him through my tears, telling him to stop, to be strong, to be the father he had always been to me, as if he was doing it on purpose, as if this were some sick joke he was playing on my mother and me.

Case Example 2

Dr. H., an anesthesiologist, was referred to me by his family doctor who worried that his patient was depressed although Dr. H. vehemently denied it. Dr. H.'s only complaint was backache. In Dr. H.'s first visit I learned that his mother and her sister were both bipolar patients on lithium; his paternal grandfather and paternal uncle had committed suicide; his father was a professional gambler who divorced his mother when Dr. H. was in medical school; Dr. H. himself had a problem with gambling, with losses in the thousands of dollars over 20 years of medical practice; his wife was attending Gamblers Anonymous for support; the family had made several moves over the years, all downward socioeconomically; Dr. H. had never been on the staff of a hospital more than 5 years; of his five children, three had severe academic and behavioral problems in school; Dr. H. himself frequently self-medicated with Ritalin in order to get going in the morning. Although Dr. H. and his wife were emotionally estranged from each other, they were committed to remaining together and trying to preserve family integrity.

Psychiatric Illness in Family Members Themselves

When working with the families of psychiatrically impaired doctors, the clinician must consider that one or more of the family members may also be struggling with some type of psychiatric illness. In a study of 56 depressed patients followed for 2 years after discharge from the hospital, Merikangas (1984) found that 30 had psychiatrically ill spouses. She also noted that couples in which both members were ill had a significantly higher divorce rate than did couples in which only one member was ill. In the field of addictionology, codependency has now been found to be a problem in those couples in which one suffers from alcohol or other drug abuse. With a clearer understanding about genetic transmission of alcoholism and mood disorders, we are better able to watch for and treat acting-out behaviors, eating disorders, academic failure, and substance abuse in the teenagers of medical families in which one or both of the parents are psychiatrically ill.

Case Example

Dr. I. first came to see me with what I diagnosed as an adjustment disorder with anxiety and depression. She was a 36-year-old resident in family medicine who had been placed on probation because of difficult interpersonal relationships with her supervisors, nurses, and fellow residents. Because she had recently separated from her unemployed husband and she was the primary caregiver of their two children, I saw her as being quite distressed in several areas of her life. However, as our work together continued, her course was like a roller coaster. She and her husband reconciled, which seemed harmonious at first, but within 3 months Dr. I. became seriously depressed and attempted suicide. After a brief hospitalization, a trial of antidepressant medication, and a brief course of marital therapy, she was asymptomatic and doing well both at home and in her residency. Within a few weeks, her husband was apprehended for shoplifting, and Dr. I. called me in a panic. I arranged for Mr. I. to be assessed and treated by a forensic psychiatrist, who actually found him to be quite depressed. Mr. I. was started on medication and subsequently improved. This psychiatrist recommended more marital therapy, and in the course of this, Dr. and Mr. I.'s 12-year-old daughter began losing weight, refused to eat her meals, and developed a number of touching and checking rituals around the home. She was assessed by a child psychiatrist and was given a dual diagnosis of obsessive-compulsive disorder and anorexia nervosa.

Fear and Avoidance of Seeking Treatment

When the family members of a psychiatrically ill doctor are reluctant to consider treatment themselves if indicated, the dynamics may point to their feelings about their doctor-relative's diagnosis and treatment. If the doctor-relative has been very ill, seeking treatment may be frightening for them. If the person has had less than optimal care, the family members may have no faith or confidence that psychiatry can be of any help. If they, as relatives, have been ignored, shunned, or blamed, they may be reluctant as well. As noted above, there may be denial and/or a sense of stigmatization. Family scapegoating may also be operative; that is, as a group they work hard to keep the doctor-relative in a sick role so that they can perceive themselves as being fine.

Some doctors, many of whom are quite symptomatic and quite ill, present as a marital problem. This is more common in men doctors than in women. It is as if the marital route is the ticket of admission for treatment. Because they are anxious, these doctors try to deny that the therapist is a psychiatrist who does marital therapy; they prefer to see him or her as a "marital counselor." Many of my doctor-patients in this category are quite jarred when I do "doctor things" (i.e., take a medical history, do a review of systems, do a mental status exam, suggest medication).

A significant number of my male physician patients who have done extensive psychotherapy with me or who required medication for a clinical illness first came with their wives for marital therapy. Once rapport is established and they feel safe, these men can begin to look at their own personal issues and consider doing some individual therapy.

Case Example

Dr. J. and Dr. K. came together for marital therapy. They were a childless couple who had been married for 5 years and felt at a stalemate with each other about whether to have children. Both were very ambivalent about kids and quite ambivalent about each other. I learned in my individual visits with each of them that their backgrounds had been terribly deprived and chaotic. They had known each other since elementary school but only really became intimate in medical school. Both realized that they clung together in a type of mutually protective and insular pact. During the fifth conjoint visit each requested to see me alone the following week. It was during those visits that

Dr. J. told me that his wife was bulimic and had been for years and that she was too ashamed to see anyone about it. Dr. K., in her individual visit, told me that her husband was addicted to Demerol and had recently nearly been "found out" after forging a prescription at the hospital where he worked.

Psychiatrists' Reluctance to Treat Family Members of Doctors

The reluctance of psychiatrists to treat the families of psychiatrically ill doctors may be the same type of reluctance that they feel when the doctor is the patient. But as noted above, when we take a family-systems perspective, we see that other family members are at risk for problems and may themselves need help. Quite clearly much work needs to be done in this area and more psychiatrists need to become involved (Myers 1988).

It has long been known that doctor-patients and their families may arouse anxiety in the treating physician (Lipsitt 1975). There are many reasons for this. There may be a feeling of vulnerability in the treating doctor (i.e., that doctors and their families are not immune to illness). There may be a fear of contagion. In *Illness as Metaphor*, Sontag (1978) delineates this fear most eloquently:

> Although the way in which disease mystifies is set against a backdrop of new expectations, the disease itself . . . arouses thoroughly old-fashioned kinds of dread. Any disease that is treated as a mystery and acutely enough feared will be felt morally, if not literally, contagious. Contact with someone afflicted with a disease regarded as a mysterious malevolency inevitably feels like a trespass; worse like the violation of a taboo. (p. 6)

Other treating physicians may feel scrutinized by the doctor-patient or his or her family, especially if many of the family members are also doctors (Marzuk 1987), and even more so if they too are psychiatrists (Fleischer and Wissler 1985).

Some doctors shun doctor-patients and their families because they feel that these patients are demanding and will need more work (Rabin et al. 1982). Some psychiatrists fail to treat the doctor-patient as a patient; that is, they do not allow the doctor to assume "patient status." The treating physician may intellectualize with the doctor-patient or engage in "medical shoptalk," thereby avoiding the patient's problem, including his or her feelings about being a patient and being ill. Finally, some psychiatrists caring for doctor-patients and their families may have heightened sensitivity to medical questioning and a proneness to defensiveness; they may perceive criticism by the patient and family when it is not there.

When the Family Receives Less Than Optimal Care

Because physician-patients may take shortcuts to treatment or because they can make their treating doctors uncomfortable, it is not unusual for them to be underexamined and/or underdiagnosed (Philips 1983). Although many doctors receive "million-dollar" workups, this is not always what they want, and in the process of being subjected to this cutting-edge technology, the person within becomes lost. Unfortunately, many of the members of the doctor's family feel this way as well. In our quest to do a superb job, we also are very busy in our professional lives, and the families of our patients fall through the cracks. Not only do we do them a disservice when we do not set aside time for them, but we fail to appreciate the rich sociocultural context in which our patients lead their lives. In this way, we may in turn short-change the patient because our diagnostic framework and treatment strategies are too narrowly defined and rigid.

Case Example

Mr. L. was a 22-year-old second-year medical student who was referred to me by the student health service of his university. He was suffering from a near delusional belief that he had contracted AIDS from an allegedly gay man who had shared a house with him the previous summer while he was working in biological research. He had both obsessive-compulsive disorder and major depression. After a tumultuous course and worsening of his symptoms, Mr. L. responded to clomipramine, lithium, and L-tryptophan. What was most critical in this man's care was my professional involvement with his mother. Her son's illness was devastating for her: she worried constantly that he really did have AIDS and not a psychiatric illness, she worried that her son was gay (despite no evidence of this), she worried that he might have been sexually assaulted by the roommate, and she worried that she herself (as an operating room nurse) might have contracted AIDS. Despite my urging that she herself see a psychiatrist, she refused. Consequently, much of my work with her son included seeing him alone, her alone, and the two of them together. In fact, she required much more psychotherapy than he did.

Conclusion

In this chapter I have given merely an overview of the many issues that arise for families in which a doctor-member is struggling with a psychiatric disorder. I have tried to emphasize that family members are fighting stigma as much as our doctor-patients, and, in some cases, even more so. There is an enormous amount that we as psychiatrists can do, not only as clinicians in reaching out to them but also as advocates for them. Stigmatization against its psychiatrically ill members remains rampant in medicine, and we must continue to educate our colleagues about modern psychiatry and what we do. Finally, we must continue to fight stigma in other doctors and in ourselves.

It is fitting to close by returning to the affect of shame, as described by Nathanson (1987), an expert on this emotion:

> So shame is all around us, part of the air we breathe. But it is not inert, not the benign and innocent source of humor it sometimes appears to be. As therapists we can learn its layers, learn to ask the questions that draw our attention beneath the surface as we have learned to do for other affects. It can be a weapon of the most insidious sort and of variable intensity. If we ignore its effect on the lives of those who come to us for help, we misunderstand such things as their failure to improve and fall into diagnostic complacency, labeling their silence as the absence of symptoms or as petulant withdrawal, instead of seeing it as an integral part of the experience of embarrassment. We begin to understand that the diagnostic labels that make us comfortable are in themselves a source of shame to our patients, and that a patient's refusal to perform a behavioral task may be out of unrevealed embarrassment rather than obsessional stubbornness. (pp. 268–269)

References

American Psychiatric Association: Diagnostic and Statistical Manual of Mental Disorders, 3rd Edition, Revised. Washington, DC, American Psychiatric Association, 1987

Briscoe CW, Smith JB: Depression and marital turmoil. Arch Gen Psychiatry 29:811–817, 1973

Fleischer JA, Wissler A: The therapist as patient: special problems and considerations. Psychotherapy 22:587–594, 1985

Lipsitt D: The doctor as patient. Psychiatric Opinion 12:20–25, 1975

Marzuk PM: When the patient is a physician. N Engl J Med 317:1409–1411, 1987

Merikangas KR: Divorce and assortative mating among depressed patients. Am J Psychiatry 141:74–76, 1984

Myers MF: Doctors' Marriages: A Look at the Problems and Their Solutions. New York, Plenum, 1988

Nathanson DL: Shaming systems in couples, families, and institutions, in The Many Faces of Shame. Edited by Nathanson DL. New York, Guilford, 1987, pp 246–270

Philips JB III: Caring for other physicians. N Engl J Med 308:1542–1543, 1983

Rabin D, Rabin PL, Rabin R: Compounding the ordeal of ALS: isolation from my fellow physicians. N Engl J Med 307:506–509, 1982

Sontag S: Illness as Metaphor. New York, Farrar, Straus, Giroux, 1978

Will OA Jr.: The sense of shame in psychosis: random comments on shame in the psychotic experience, in The Many Faces of Shame. Edited by Nathanson DL. New York, Guilford, 1987, pp 308–317

Institutional Issues

Chapter 14

The Stigma of Mental Illness for Medical Students and Residents

Leah J. Dickstein, M.D.
Lisa D. Hinz, Ph.D.

In this chapter the authors consider the sociocultural, personal, situational, and professional factors that are integral to the stigma of mental illness for medical students and residents, and examine the consequent difficulties faced by students and residents in referring themselves for psychiatric treatment. The high social status of physicians, the denial and suppression of emotions that characterize medical students, and the medical profession's emphasis on patients' needs rather than one's own needs make it difficult for medical students and residents to acknowledge their need for treatment.

Solutions and recommendations for combating stigma are presented. They include faculty sharing their own family histories of mental illness, ongoing programs that focus on stress and distress, visible support groups, emphasis on the confidentiality of psychiatric treatment, and student exposure to outpatients with less dramatic problems such as depression and anxiety. Teachers, mentors, and therapists must encourage, guide, and support students in their quest for appropriate, available treatment without negative consequences.

Although in the past decade psychiatric illness has become more legitimate in the eyes of the public, routinely discussed in the media, more an integral part of general medicine, and increasingly mainstream for the health insurance industry, in labs, lecture halls, lounges, study areas, residents' offices, and hallways, many medical students and residents remain reluctant to acknowledge their illness to peers and professors and to seek appropriate psychiatric treatment. In the same vein, their peers and attending physicians are reluctant to confront the students and residents about recommending the latter seek help. This reluctance is based upon sociocultural, personal, situational, and professional reasons, and is, in large measure, related to the unique, excessive, and dangerous stigma attached by most medical professionals to their own and their colleagues' mental illness.

What medical students and residents have learned and experienced at conscious and, more likely, unconscious levels about mental illness in their premedical lifetimes has certainly led them to expect and accept stigma as an integral part of the process by which a mentally ill person first recognizes his or her illness and the need for treatment, and consequently searches for involvement in appropriate therapy. Variations on this attitude, along with certain personality traits, can be considered the personal factors that contribute to the stigmatization of mental illness for medical students and residents and that result in their reluctance to seek psychiatric help. Reluctance to approach their own and others' illness, especially mental illness, can also be attributed to sociocultural myths and expectations related to physician status; to situational factors related to premedical education, medical school, and residency training; and finally to factors associated with the medical profession as it has developed in the United States. Each of these factors—sociocultural, personal, situational, and professional—will be discussed, because each is considered to be integral to the stigma of mental illness for medical students and residents.

Sociocultural Factors

The American public considers physicians to be at the top of the country's occupational hierarchy. Having "made it" to the top, physicians are assumed to be emotionally stable, and are even looked upon with a kind of hero worship (Arnstein 1986; Kosch 1986). Some would go so far as to say that in our increasingly technological society, physicians, with their specialized knowledge of science and its modern technological trappings, have replaced the clergy as America's counselors and confessors (Kosch 1986). People expect their physicians to be available and healthy. Any physician's request for help is seen as eroding the public's expectation and the physician's personal image of self-sufficiency (Roeske 1986). In addition, the physician's status (beginning with premedical studies and continuing in increasing amounts with more advanced training) promotes distance from former personal and societal norms and values and results in physicians being placed on a pedestal (Dickstein 1986; Levin 1988). Thus, distance from society's norms for behavior and a hero-like status exacerbate the stigma of mental illness for medical students and residents and make it exceedingly difficult for them to ask for psychiatric help.

Even if a medical student or resident did decide to seek psychiatric treatment, the insurance coverage for mental disorders available to them is often shameful (e.g., three inpatient days and $500 for outpatient care per year). Having to respond to questions about psychiatric treatment and emotional illness on medical licensure applications is a reality in many states and a current agenda item for the American Psychiatric Association's Committee on Medical Student Education. The stigma experienced by public figures and recounted by the media concerning mental illness fuels residents' fears that they will be unable to practice medicine if their psychiatric treatment becomes known in their communities. These fears are fueled not only by licensure problems but also by the loss of status and resulting lack of referrals from colleagues who have lost trust in and respect for them.

Personal Factors

The same personality traits that help ambitious students gain admission to medical school can predispose them later to be especially susceptible to the effects of stigma surrounding mental illness. For example, most authors mention that the preferred defense mechanisms of medical students and residents are denial, repression, and displacement of feelings (Doyle 1983; Levin 1988; Lohr and Engbring 1988; Pfifferling 1986; Roeske 1986; Shapiro et al. 1987; Vitalino et al. 1989). Workaholism, guilt, and self-denial begin during premedical studies as students deny themselves normal pleasures and continue studying because of the inordinate guilt and fear motivating them. For example, they might think, "Someone who studied harder might get that enviable position in medical school!" Self-denial continues throughout medical school and residency training as students are taught to deny their own needs in the service of their patients (Grouse 1981; Pfifferling 1986). Defensive denial is often used by medical students and residents to tell themselves that they are doing better than they really are (Pfifferling 1986). Denial of illness in themselves and in their families is extremely vigorous among medical students and trainees. Many who finally enter treatment speak about striving for success in school during their developmental years as a means of emotional survival and avoidance of the truth about the chronic problems in themselves and in their families.

Self-esteem remains excessively tied to academic achievement; in medical school and residency this often means successfully mastering enormous amounts of course material. However, students commonly find that they cannot master the tremendous volume of medical school material required with the ease with which they once mastered coursework prior to medical school. Consequently, self-esteem plummets, and anxiety or a depressive reaction may follow. Medical students too often see themselves as so obedient, passive, and self-doubting that they do not know when to ask for help (or give it) when it is needed (Kosch 1986). The end result is emotional isolation characterized by the fact that a large number of medical students and residents suffer from self-doubt and feelings of inadequacy; yet most are unaware that these feelings are not unique or that they are not a sign of weakness or incompetency (Coombs and Fawzy 1986; Kosch 1986).

Students and residents, to the point in their lives at which they admit to being mentally ill, have rarely felt vulnerable; rather they have been the achievers, the all-American high school and college success stories. They, the ones voted most likely to succeed, believed success neither included nor permitted psychiatric illness. By identifying themselves as patients they simultaneously begin to doubt all of their competencies—both personal and professional. They stigmatize and isolate themselves as they ashamedly, angrily, and fearfully reject themselves; they perceive potential rejection from others often where it does not exist. Clearly for these students and residents self-stigmatization is the most overwhelming discrimination of all. Such isolation and self-stigmatization unfortunately ensure that even if medical students do feel the need for psychiatric help they will not ask for it. There is a tendency among these students to deny psychological conflicts or to have these conflicts be expressed as physical illness (Doyle 1983). However, physical illnesses often go untreated; 70% of physicians do not schedule regular physical exams, and more than 60% do not even have a personal physician (Pfifferling 1986).

Their professional education to date has not affected the degree of shame that medical students and residents feel about the possibility of becoming a psychiatric patient. For example, one student adamantly and steadfastly refused a trial of antidepressant medication that was obviously indicated and finally conceded after 10 years of intermittent psychotherapy. At that point he was healthy enough to state that he had fought medication because to him it represented the ultimate step that would legitimize his stigma as a psychiatric patient.

Others become angry at developing psychiatric symptoms that finally force them to seek treatment, but they often have difficulty verbalizing this anger. Their anger includes having to break away from classes, rounds, clinics, surgery, and studying to keep individual appointments and group sessions. They need time and the development of trust in themselves and in their therapists to admit to their assumed and self-assigned guilt over having, they believe, caused their illness through personal weakness and inadequacy. They are angry at the shame that they feel about themselves being psychiatrically ill and about their fears of never recovering and of rejection by significant others, family, friends, peers, and teachers.

Situational Factors

Situational factors associated with medical school and residency training increase the stigma of mental illness and make it difficult for students and residents to seek psychiatric treatment. These factors include enormous time commitments and clinical responsibilities. Schedules too often are set on service, not on educational needs, and students receive the tacit message that they are considered last (Aach et al. 1988). Aside from requiring a large amount of time, medical school and residency training require tremendous amounts of energy and commitment both in and outside of the hospital. Training is undoubtedly stressful (Aach et al. 1988; Levin 1988; Lohr and Engbring 1988; Pfifferling 1986); one author went so far as to compare the internship to yearlong fraternity hazing (Cousins 1981).

More important than the actual stress caused by medical training is the management of that stress. Unfortunately, training most commonly models overwork and denial of stress (Pfifferling 1986). Older physicians who are trainees' first role models may not be influenced by the same stress as students (e.g., starting a career, marriage, and family all at the same time), or if they are under stress they do not feel free to talk about it (Levin 1988). Medical training models the "man of steel" (Levin 1988) or "white knight" (Dickstein 1986) approach to stress: Men continue to deny emotional pain and psychiatric symptomatology and remain in psychological control until their spouses or significant others leave them, at which time the professional men decompensate, often to severe, incapacitating depression and suicidal states. But until that point, medical students and residents are taught to deny their own needs (including their often escalating stress levels) and instead attend only to their patients' needs (Grouse 1981).

Medical schools and residency programs frequently fail to recognize the diminishing returns of too much stress (Levin 1988). In addition, they also fail to take into account that optimal levels of stress differ for different people (Aach et al. 1988). Instead, training programs seem to adhere to the "pathology model" of training stress (Levin 1988, p. 120) in which all stress experienced by medical students and residents is seen as illness or weakness. Such "illnesses" have been named, for example, "medical student disease" and "house officer stress syndrome" (Arnstein 1986; Small et al. 1969), and the application of these labels can be used to call into question trainees' "fitness" to practice medicine (Arnstein 1986; Kosch 1986; Levin 1988). Students and residents may be reluctant to ask for help in such an atmosphere because they fear automatic dismissal or some other equally unpleasant consequence.

From their very first medical school lectures, students observe an unfortunate attitude prevalent in a sizable number of their teachers. A large percentage of these students have heard their professors, attendings, and residents speak indiscreetly about mentally ill patients in less than respectful terms, divulging patients' identities and personal information as well as revealing professional attitudes filled with ignorance, repugnance, hopelessness, disinterest, fear, and stigma about those "psych patients." (One must wonder if attitudes might be different if someone were diagnosed with "mental hypertension" rather than with schizophrenia, or with "chronic hyposerotoninemia of the locus coeruleus" rather than with depression.) Students also have observed during their clinical rotations that recommendations for psychiatric consultations, although commonly requested, may be incompletely followed up or ignored. Students imitate faculty members' ways of coping and soon are seen as being overworked and as using sarcasm about their undesirable patients as a method of coping (Roy et al. 1988).

Concerns about confidentiality are among the most important situational factors involved in students' hesitation to refer themselves for psychiatric services (Aach et al. 1988; Arnstein 1986; Doyle 1983). In a 1989 national survey of women residents in all specialties and of their experiences with stress, it was found that 92% with admitted medical illness sought treatment, whereas only 73% with acknowledged emotional illness did so (Dickstein and Bachelor 1989). Was concern about stigma a factor in the lower percent seeking mental health treatment? The unusually small and confined medical school and university hospital community are settings ripe and rife for the relaying of rumors designed to instigate terror, shame, and self-doubt in those who are vulnerable. Rumors also circulate that dismissal is possible for trainees as well as for students with psychiatric illness. Fear that their confidentiality will be broken and their personal distress circulated throughout the school/hospital certainly prevents some medical students from requesting the help that they need.

Professional Factors

Medicine has traditionally been a male-dominated profession in which the expression of feelings is perceived as being weak and unprofessional. Stress reactions by trainees are taken as proof that they were not cut out for the profession in the first place (Kosch 1986). Women medical students and residents are more likely than men to admit feeling the pressure and stigma (Dickstein et al. 1989, 1990; Linn and Zeppa 1984; Lloyd 1983; Lloyd and Gartell 1984) and believe that they must be twice as good as men in order to be considered adequate (Hawk and Scott 1986). Thus women are probably inhibited from asking for help because they are afraid of exposing their twofold "weakness": being female and needing psychiatric help.

Preferred coping mechanisms are suppression and intellectualization of emotions (Coombs and Fawzy 1986; Hawk and Scott 1986). Within the still male-dominated medical system, the "basic" or "hard" sciences such as chemistry and biology are valued over "soft" ones such as behavioral sciences. The system idealizes technology and science over other disciplines (Kosch 1986; Pfifferling 1986). The implicit and often explicit message given to trainees is that psychiatry is not "scientific" enough to be a highly valued specialty in medicine (Doyle 1983; Singer et al. 1986; Yager et al. 1982). In fact, psychiatry is rated as one of the low-status medical specialties by an overwhelming proportion of medical students (Das and Chandrasena 1988; Doyle 1983; Yager et al. 1982), and other departments are perceived as being critical of psychiatry (Das and Chandrasena 1988).

During behavioral science lectures on human development, students are confronted with genetic predispositions to frightening diseases without current permanent cure: schizophrenia, personality disorders, the problem of suicide, and the effects that alcohol wreaks on families as well as on its victims. They either automatically distance themselves from even passing thoughts that they might someday suffer from these illnesses, or, already having experienced these disorders in themselves or their families, they slink down in their seats with shame, sadness, and apprehension. In other lectures they also hear about chronic illnesses such as hypertension and diabetes with which they or their families may be afflicted, but these diseases are not ones students or society connect to stigmatization.

It is quite different with mental illness. For example, in 1 month three medical students entered therapy with a variety of personal and marital problems. These students verbalized and acknowledged, apparently for the first time in their lives, the fact that one of their parents suffered from alcoholism and that their early milieu was a dysfunctional family. They all initially denied what they now admitted to, and needed much support, education, and challenge to accept what they felt as the stigma of this illness of chemical dependency probably as part of a dual diagnosis. One student recounted that she had seen our notice for an Adult Children of Alcoholics group on campus and had thought seriously about going, but could not get herself to do so. She would have continued to avoid therapy as long as she could, but "broke down" uncontrollably in conversation with a sensitive teacher who referred her for treatment. She then attempted to deny problems, took a "flight into health" after two sessions, and was confronted about this when it was obvious she had not yet truly entered treatment. Finally, she admitted that she was ashamed to "make her problems public," in a group or even in individual psychotherapy. Additionally she verbalized her worry that the therapist "had more important things to do than to help [her]." A male medical student entered therapy because his wife had decided to seek a divorce and he felt overwhelmed and began abusing alcohol. The third student complained of depression and helplessness. She had recently discovered her husband's infidelity and felt suicidal.

Because patients suffering from psychotic disorders are referred for psychiatric evaluation, but less disturbed patients are not, students and residents learn a biased referral attitude from faculty (Rudsill et al. 1989). Therefore, trainees might be less likely to refer themselves for treatment if they do not perceive themselves as being acutely psychotic. In addition, the efficacy of psychiatric treatment often has not been demonstrated to students in their behavioral science courses and clinical clerkships (Doyle 1983; Singer et al. 1986; Yager et al. 1982). Students are exposed to severe inpatient psychopathology and, often because of decreasing hospital stays, insurance coverage, and length of rotations, do not follow patients long enough to see significant changes resulting from psychiatric treatment (Yager et al. 1982). Thus, in the medical profession negative attitudes toward psychiatry, psychiatric patients, and psychiatric treatment greatly contribute to the stigmatization of those with mental illness and further impede medical students and residents from seeking personal treatment.

Langsley (1983) mentions the "age old stigma" (p. ix) attached to mental illness in the medical profession. Physicians do not want to become ill, especially mentally ill; but if they do, they are admonished to diagnose and heal themselves (Doyle 1983). Because of the attitude of professional courtesy, many physicians believe that they do not need comprehensive medical plans, especially for psychiatric treatment. However, when it actually comes down to asking for professional courtesy, most physicians do not do so because they do not want to bother their colleagues (Pfifferling 1986; Robinowitz 1983; Scheiber and Doyle 1983). Thus their many illnesses, including psychiatric ones, go untreated.

Some students and residents decide to seek "counseling" with other mental health professionals—social workers, psychologists, their religious leaders, pastoral counselors, and the myriad assortment of therapists—rather than be seen by a psychiatrist even when vegetative and mental status signs of needing medication are identified. If a psychiatrist has judged their psychological, emotional, or "mental" problem not to be organically based, then seeing a professional trained in another discipline is fine. However, this is usually not the case. In fact, we must all become aware, if we are not already, that many administrators (Ph.D. and M.D. faculty) and many even in our own departments refer, suggest, direct, advise, and warn students and residents to seek nonpsychiatric treatment because seeking psychiatric care would blemish their academic and professional records, complicate future medical insurance and state licensing procedures, and affect how important others would think about them if they were to discover that the students and residents had been seen professionally by a psychiatrist!

State medical societies have set up impaired physician committees that are designed to identify, refer, and help secure treatment for physicians with emotional problems. However, the prevailing attitude in the medical profession is that these committees are conducting searches akin to witch-hunts in which impaired physicians are sought out and punished (Lohr and Engbring 1988). Clearly this attitude must be addressed and changed if the stigma surrounding mental illness for physicians is to be effectively reduced.

Recommendations for Combating Stigma

To help reduce the stigma surrounding physician impairment and mental illness, sociocultural, professional, situational, and personal factors must be confronted. The factors on which we as educators can most greatly have an impact are those related to medical education and training. Perhaps by focusing our efforts on training situations, we can eventually influence professional and sociocultural factors. Personal factors must be addressed by educators who come into contact with and serve as role models for medical students and residents. Faculty must dare to take the risk of sharing information about their own family histories of mental illness. By our own example—this will be the real reason that students and residents begin to overcome their stigma toward mental illness. Educators must realize (and hopefully teach) that in order to care for others we must first care for ourselves (Mentink and Scott 1986; Shapiro et al. 1987). In addition, faculty must develop and implement specific guidelines and procedures to help students and residents in difficulty (Shapiro et al. 1987; Urbach and Levenson 1988; Wald and Miller 1982).

Physicians characteristically have been reluctant to confront psychological distress, especially distress perceived as being caused by the medical system itself (Arnstein 1986). However, in order to effectively reduce the stigma surrounding psychological disorders, the issues of stress and distress must be openly discussed and normalized (Shapiro et al. 1987). This open discussion should begin at orientation and continue throughout training; it should include information about wellness, techniques for stress management, and encouragement to seek treatment when needed (Dickstein and Elkes 1986; Mentink and Scott 1986). Shapiro and her colleagues (1987) suggested that spouses and significant others should be involved in ongoing discussions of medical student and resident distress because they are likely to be the first ones to be affected by it.

In addition to normalizing the stress and distress involved in medical training through informational lectures, there should be available visible in-house support groups (e.g., Dickstein 1982) that allow trainees or their significant others a chance to find out that their feelings of self-doubt and inadequacy are shared by many and that these feelings are not a sign of weakness. Hopefully such sharing will reduce the emotional isolation felt by so many medical students and residents and make it easier for them to ask for more formal psychiatric treatment if needed.

Students and residents must repeatedly be assured by hospital and school policy, as well as by faculty behavior, that their confidentiality will be respected if they do seek psychiatric treatment. Better insurance coverage for mental disorders and substance abuse treatment will give the message that seeking treatment for these disorders is acceptable and encouraged. If possible, the distressed trainee should be reassured that seeking treatment or even taking a leave of absence will not lead to detrimental consequences for future medical training or the practice of medicine. Reassurance is more likely to be felt if faculty construct a system for dealing with distressed students and residents that is humane and objective as well as confidential (Shapiro et al. 1987).

The stigma of mental illness can be effectively combated in the classroom. One way to reduce stigma would be to increase the status of psychiatry in the eyes of medical students. In order to do this it clearly must be demonstrated that psychiatry has considerable scientific merit, that psychiatric treatments are effective, and that psychiatrists have a unique role as mental health professionals (Das and Chandrasena 1988; Doyle 1983; Singer et al. 1986). Singer and colleagues (1986) suggest that assigning courses in the behavioral sciences to psychiatrist-instructors is necessary to show students how psychiatry is a unique mental health profession.

In our lectures during all years of medical education we should certainly teach about psychoses, but we should emphasize what is usually, because of lack of time, glossed over: the less dramatic problems that outpatients bring to treatment (e.g., depression, anxiety, psychosomatic and personality disorders) that constitute the majority of disorders that nonpsychiatrist physicians will see and diagnose—that is, if we teach them how to do so rather than leaving them unprepared and therefore frustrated with so-called uncooperative, "chronic" patients. Not understanding the psychiatric aspects of their patients can lead untrained physicians to stigmatize all mentally ill persons, including themselves. We should start our teaching with the most treatable patients—that in itself will help decrease the problem of stigma.

Students and residents should be given well-disguised examples of impaired medical students and residents from many years past to repeatedly impress the fact that it is legitimate and safe to be mentally ill, to receive treatment, and to recover. They should have at their disposal well-known options of treatment sites, inpatient and outpatient, locally and elsewhere. They will enter treatment and refer their peers if they believe it is safe. This process will escalate constructively and in an ongoing student "generation-to-generation" manner through the rumor mill—but for good purposes rather than because of fear and misinformation.

We should send students off independently to assume responsibilities for psychiatric patients only after they have worked at our sides, watched us, and observed our attitudes toward psychiatric illness and psychiatric patients. Students should be actively taught to treat the psychiatric patient as a whole person, to ask all of the appropriate questions, and to obtain complete medical histories before thinking about prescribing a psychotropic medication.

Educating all students and residents in a theoretical mode is fine and highly recommended, but to reach into the core of their (and our) fears and defenses about mental illness, we must be creative. We believe that assigning every student to a family with a mentally ill member the first week of medical school and requiring that the student follow the family for 4 years would offer the opportunity to gain more exposure to outpatient as well as inpatient treatment, and to see the positive effects of psychiatric treatment over time. We know that many junior students obtain better medical, including psychiatric, histories because they make and have the time to spend with their patients. Reasonable time requirements over a 4-year block would facilitate the reduction of the power of psychiatric stigma for students as they become appropriately involved with recovering and relapsing assigned individuals and their support systems.

Conclusion

The stigma of mental illness for physicians stems from factors related to the sociocultural status of physicians and from the denial and suppression of emotions characteristic of premedical students that is reinforced throughout medical training. The medical profession is built on the belief that to express feelings is weak and that one's own needs should be denied and only patients' needs met. Within the medical profession psychiatry is looked upon with a mixture of contempt, fear, and awe; it is seen as less scientific and of lower status than other medical specialties.

In order to reduce the stigma surrounding mental illness that makes it difficult for physicians to refer themselves and their colleagues for psychiatric treatment, all of these factors—sociocultural, professional, personal, and situational—must be addressed. The easiest way to confront the stigma of mental illness and psychiatric treatment is by addressing it directly in classrooms and clerkships. However, in order to do this, educators must first examine their own attitudes and values so that they can provide an open, nonjudgmental atmosphere for an ongoing and humane dialogue on medical training distress and stigma.

Paul Fink's brilliant and timely decision to focus on "Overcoming the Stigma of Psychiatry" at the 1989 annual meeting of the American Psychiatric Association clearly refers to students and residents as patients and professionals, and we, their teachers, mentors, and therapists, must encourage, guide, and support them in their quest for appropriate, available, indicated treatment without negative consequences.

References

Aach RD, Cooney TG, Girard DE, et al: Stress and impairment during residency training: strategies for reduction, identification, and management. Ann Intern Med 109:54–61, 1988

Arnstein RL: Emotional problems of medical students. Am J Psychiatry 143:1422–1423, 1986

Coombs RH, Fawzy FI: The impaired-physician syndrome: a developmental perspective, in Heal Thyself: The Health of Health Care Professionals. Edited by Scott CD, Hawk J. New York, Brunner/Mazel, 1986, pp 44–55

Cousins N: Internship: preparation or hazing? JAMA 245:277, 1981

Das MP, Chandrasena RD: Medical students' attitudes towards psychiatry. Can J Psychiatry 33:783–787, 1988

Dickstein LJ: The student hour: a support group for freshmen medical students. J Am Coll Health 31:131–132, 1982

Dickstein LJ: Social change and dependency in university men: the white knight complex unresolved. Journal of College Student Psychotherapy 1:31–41, 1986

Dickstein LJ, Elkes J: A health awareness workshop: enhancing coping skills in medical students, in Heal Thyself: The Health of Health Care Professionals. Edited by Scott CD, Hawk J. New York, Brunner/Mazel, 1986, pp 269–281

Dickstein LJ, Batchelor A, Stephenson J: Stress and women residents: national survey results. Paper presented at the American Medical Women's Association, Los Angeles, CA, October 1989

Dickstein LJ, Stephenson J, Hinz LD: Role strain as a factor in medical student impairment: implications for intervention strategies. Acad Med 65:588–593, 1990

Doyle BB: Responsibility, confidentiality, and the psychiatrically ill physician, in The Impaired Physician. Edited by Scheiber SC, Doyle BB. New York, Plenum, 1983, pp 125–136

Grouse LD (ed): Internship: physicians respond to Norman Cousins. JAMA 246:2141–2144, 1981

Hawk J, Scott CD: A case of family medicine: sources of stress in residents and physicians in practice, in Heal Thyself: The Health of Health Care Professionals. Edited by Scott CD, Hawk J. New York, Brunner/Mazel, 1986, pp 71–85

Kosch SG: Physicians, stress, and family life: a systematic view, in Heal Thyself: The Health of Health Care Professionals. Edited by Scott CD, Hawk J. New York, Brunner/Mazel, 1986, pp 110–133

Langsley D: Foreword to The Impaired Physician. Edited by Scheiber SC, Doyle BB. New York, Plenum, 1983, pp 9–10

Levin R: Beyond "the men of steel": the origins and significance of house staff training stress. Gen Hosp Psychiatry 10:114–121, 1988

Linn BS, Zeppa R: Stress in junior medical students: relationship to personality and performance. Journal of Medical Education 59:7–12, 1984

Lloyd C: Sex differences in medical students requesting psychiatric intervention. J Nerv Ment Dis 171:535–545, 1983

Lloyd C, Gartell NK: Psychiatric symptoms in medical students. Compr Psychiatry 25:552–565, 1984

Lohr KM, Engbring NH: Institution-wide program for impaired residents at a major teaching hospital. Journal of Medical Education 63:182–189, 1988

Mentink J, Scott CD: Implementing a self-care curriculum, in Heal Thyself: The Health of Health Care Professionals. Edited by Scott CD, Hawk J. New York, Brunner/Mazel, 1986, pp 235–256

Pfifferling JH: Cultural antecedents promoting professional impairment, in Heal Thyself: The Health of Health Care Professionals. Edited by Scott CD, Hawk J. New York, Brunner/Mazel, 1986, pp 3–18

Robinowitz CB: The physician as a patient, in The Impaired Physician. Edited by Scheiber SC, Doyle BB. New York, Plenum, 1983, pp 137-146

Roeske NCA: Risk factors: predictable hazards of a health career, in Heal Thyself: The Health of Health Care Professionals. Edited by Scott CD, Hawk J. New York, Brunner/Mazel, 1986, pp 56-70

Roy RJ, Barret WD, Blossom NH, et al: Resident mental health: a resource pamphlet for residents and program directors. American Academy of Family Physicians, Committee on Mental Health, Kansas City, MO, 1988

Rudsill JR, Painter AF, Rodenhauer P, et al: Family physicians and referral for psychotherapy. Int J Psychiatry Med 19:249-262, 1989

Scheiber SC, Doyle BB (eds): The Impaired Physician. New York, Plenum, 1983

Shapiro J, Prislin MD, Larsen KM, et al: Working with the resident in difficulty. Fam Med 19:360-375, 1987

Singer P, Dornbush RL, Brownstein EJ, et al: Undergraduate psychiatric education and attitudes of medical students towards psychiatry. Compr Psychiatry 27:14-20, 1986

Small IF, Small JG, Assue CM, et al: Fate of the mentally ill physician. Am J Psychiatry 125:133-134, 1969

Urbach J, Levenson JL: Graduate medical education faces housestaff stress: institutional dynamics and group processes. Psychiatr Q 59:37-46, 1988

Vitalino PP, Maiuro RD, Russo J, et al: Medical student distress: a longitudinal study. J Nerv Ment Dis 177:70-76, 1989

Wall HP, Miller MJ: The Aid to Impaired Medical Students (AIMS) Program. Presented at the University of Tennessee-Memphis, 1982

Yager J, Lamotte K, Nielsen A III, et al: Medical students' evaluation of psychiatry: a cross-country comparison. Am J Psychiatry 139:1003-1009, 1982

Chapter 15

Societal Factors in the Problems Faced by Deinstitutionalized Psychiatric Patients

Amerigo Farina, Ph.D.
Jeffrey D. Fisher, Ph.D.
Edward H. Fischer, Ph.D.

In this chapter the authors examine deinstitutionalization, a movement that has been revolutionizing the care and treatment of psychiatric patients in the United States and elsewhere. Although deinstitutionalization has had both successes and failures, the focus here is on the difficulties encountered by discharged patients in fitting back into society. Consequently, the authors present a view that is gloomy to an unwarranted degree unless the reader bears in mind that there are successes not herein considered.

Farina, Fisher, and Fischer identify three general factors that may underlie the problems of deinstitutionalization: 1) stigmatization of this population by society, 2) the reaction of the deinstitutionalized population to being stigmatized, and 3) the objective characteristics of the discharged patient population. The authors indicate how these factors make the problems encountered by deinstitutionalization more understandable.

Deinstitutionalization is a development that has revolutionized the mental health field in the United States and elsewhere. A major aim of the movement has been to take psychiatric patients out of large institutions and return them to the community, where, with the aid of planned facilities such as group homes, they are expected to lead a more normal life. Generally, opinions were strongly in favor of deinstitutionalization, and it was implemented with dramatic results. For example, in the state of Massachusetts there were 23,000 patients in state mental hospitals in 1965. By 1985, that number had been reduced to a mere 2,000 according to the *Boston Sunday Globe* of March 10, 1985 (Nickerson 1985). But, even though most people concerned with this, ourselves included, still consider deinstitutionalization a good idea, with the passage of time it has become apparent that this movement is encountering serious problems. A major one is that a proportion of discharged patients do not fit back into the community and instead survive in a pitiful and hazardous manner at the margins of society. The most frequently cited (and possibly related) reasons for this problem appear to be the following. First, inadequate preparation in the community has been made to receive the expatients and to promote their reintegration into society. Group homes, job placement and training facilities, and needed advisors and coordinators have not been made available. Second, the community stigmatizes former mental patients. Because these patients are viewed as blemished and not accepted on their merits, the readjustment process is made much more difficult than it might otherwise be.

Unquestionably both factors play a role, as do many other factors that have also been cited. Our interest, however, is centered on the second factor, stigma. In what follows we first briefly consider the evidence indicating the problems that the issue of deinstitutionalization has encountered. Specifically, a sizeable number of former psychiatric patients are living in the community under extremely difficult conditions. We then review pertinent research on stigma, primarily that concerned with mental disorders. We believe that research makes the problems encountered in reintegrating discharged patients into the community more understandable, and it might conceivably suggest procedures for making deinstitutionalization a better and less painful process for all involved.

Problems Encountered by Deinstitutionalized Psychiatric Patients

Some of the information indicating problems in returning patients to the community comes from formal research. A very high number of discharged patients are unemployed, even after being in the community for 1 year (e.g., Anthony et al. 1972; Lamb and Goertzel 1977; Pepper et al. 1981). It appears that not more than one-third of them are employed, and as many as 85% have been reported as not being engaged in any paid work. Work is a highly important factor in determining social status for men and, increasingly, for women. Of course, if there is no income the individual can face very severe practical problems such as not having food or housing. Clearly the unemployment figures indicate that the discharged patients are not assuming a role that is critically important in the community. Many of the returnees also fail to do basic day-to-day activities such as shop for needed supplies. According to a study reported by Kiesler and Sibulkin (1987), 30% were unable or unwilling to use available transportation, 31% did not maintain personal hygiene, and 40% to 50% did not go shopping, prepare meals, or maintain an adequate diet unless, in each instance, someone assisted them. Half or more could not manage available funds, use transportation on unfamiliar routes, or take prescribed medication. Moreover, the same authors reported that from about one-fifth to one-third of deinstitutionalized patients caused complaints from neighbors, engaged in bizarre behavior, had trouble at work or school, or exhibited temper tantrums.

In addition to the foregoing systematic studies, the mass media have given a great deal of attention to this problem. Of course, reports in newspapers, television, and radio may, at times, be biased and also can easily be selected to support a variety of positions. Nevertheless, much relevant information is available from those sources that does not seem to be provided by research: this information presents a picture of deinstitutionalized patients that is quite gloomy. A *Boston Sunday Globe* article (Nickerson 1985) quotes the then-president of the American Psychiatric Association (APA), John A. Talbott, M.D., as follows: "I'm trying to reform the mental health system; we've gone from atrocious to awful" (p. 1). The reporter who wrote the article, Colin Nickerson, continues: "As a result (of new policies), tens of thousands of desperately ill individuals have wound up in shelters for the homeless or jail; tens of thousands more languish, forgotten, in rooming houses or in rest homes where the only 'therapy' is a droning TV set." And in an article published in the *Hartford Courant* in 1986, E. Fuller Torrey, a Washington research psychiatrist, begins:

> Has deinstitutionalization been a failure? Take a walk through the parks of the city—any city—and decide for yourself. Count the number of disturbed individuals chatting amiably to the air, gesticulating wildly to the clouds or standing mute in the shadows of decaying buildings like 20th century gargoyles. These mentally ill individuals were not part of our landscape 25 years ago before we started to empty state mental hospitals.

Numerous events reported in the mass media substantiate these pessimistic evaluations. Moreover, the reports clearly indicate that some members of the community do not want former psychiatric patients living among them. First of all, this source of information indicates that many deinstitutionalized people are homeless. There is no way to tell exactly what proportion of homeless people are former patients, nor even how many homeless people there are at any given time. We can quickly see why we lack precise figures regarding this if we consider, as an example, the procedures the city of Boston has had to follow in trying to obtain such information. In an article in the *Hartford Courant* in 1988 (February 20; C8), the author states that during the month of February an attempt was made in Boston to determine how many homeless people were in that city. After taking a census of all those in shelters provided by the city one night, the following night 117 volunteers proceeded after midnight to walk nearly every street in Boston and to search every nook that could serve as a shelter for someone. Even this compulsive method, with the aid of flashlights, walkie-talkies, and police escorts, would not succeed. According to one of the volunteers, "We still don't get all the homeless. There are people hidden away in buildings we'll just never find."

However, enough is known to make it obvious that many discharged patients are homeless and are otherwise in dire circumstances. Communities, even large cities, seem overwhelmed and unable to care for these individuals. Thus, on May 21, 1982, a New York radio station, WCBS, reported that New York City was seeking aid from the state so that it could provide housing for 6,000 discharged psychiatric patients. And on November 1, 1986, the "CBS Evening News" reported a similar occurrence at the national level. Federal funds in the sum of $100 million were slated to be distributed to seven cities to provide shelters for homeless individuals who were there because of deinstitutionalization. The program also reported that an estimated 20% to 50% of all homeless individuals are former psychiatric patients. A similar proportion, 40%, was the estimate given on the "NBC Nightly News" on April 12, 1987.

The situation for some of these former patients is so bad that a disproportionately large percentage die, according to a report by Dr. Donald W. Black, a psychiatrist at the University of Iowa Hospital and Clinics, Iowa City. Even if enough shelter space were to be made available to accommodate all expatients, that would not eliminate the problem, because some of the individuals are disturbed and require close supervision. A number of them are being placed in jails, according to a WGBH broadcast from Boston (May 21, 1980). Other efforts to deal with the problem have included attempts to enact laws making it more difficult to discharge psychiatric patients from institutions. Congressman Stewart B. McKinney of Connecticut introduced a bill in the House of Representatives that calls for such a law (*Hartford Courant*, November 11, 1983). And the Connecticut Hospital Association was reported to be considering suing the State of Connecticut to force it to increase the number of beds in its mental hospitals (Rhinelander *Hartford Courant* 1983).

The mass media also make it obvious that community resistance to aspects of deinstitutionalization is strong and quite effective. This, of course, is consistent with the frequent mention of stigma as one of the causes of the problems posed by deinstitutionalization. In an article in the *New York Times* entitled "Resistance Rises to Group Homes for Mental Cases," Clifford D. May (1986) summarized what he learned from his investigation: "To many residents of [communities containing group homes], mainstreaming means the threat of falling property values, diminished personal security, and more frequent encounters with the disabled than they might wish" (p. 1). An event that occurred in Greenwich, Connecticut, provides a vivid illustration of the views of expatients held in some quarters. A "halfway house for mentally ill patients" was established in that town, and residents on the same street asked the Greenwich Board of Tax Review to reduce the property assessment on their houses. They claimed the presence of the halfway house would make selling their homes more difficult. The Board granted the complaining homeowners reductions ranging from $2,960 to $10,270 (Megan *Hartford Courant* 1985). What transpired in Greenwich appears to be very unusual and was denounced by sundry officials including the Connecticut Attorney General and First Selectman of Greenwich. However, resistance to the establishment of community facilities for discharged mental patients is far from unusual. The following information given to a *Hartford Courant* reporter in 1986 by Audrey M. Worrell, who was then Mental Health Commissioner for the State of Connecticut, illustrates this point. There were 14 group homes in Connecticut at that time. For seven of these, community resistance had been encountered in the form of either "local zoning actions or regulatory delays." At least eight proposed homes did not open because of local hostility or "the perception that community resistance could not be overcome." Also, three group homes were at that time under construction, and two of these had met with opposition.

Stigma Research

Research on stigma that bears on the problems encountered in returning psychiatric patients to the community will now be reviewed. First, we will examine society's disposition to see people who have had psychiatric problems as being seriously blemished and to treat them differently and often less favorably. We will then review studies showing that this social stigma has an adverse effect on the stigmatized *in addition* to the direct impact of the negative social actions (e.g., denying work to former mental patients). Finally, research focusing on some objective characteristics of deinstitutionalized patients will be considered. As will be shown, these characteristics, such as deficiencies in social skills, evidently act to make the reintegration process more difficult.

A Stigmatizing Society

After more than a quarter of a century of systematic study, we can now be quite sure of how the public feels about people with mental disorders (Nunnally 1961). Such individuals are typically viewed in a highly negative way. Furthermore, the public's feelings and comportment toward afflicted persons do not seem to be improving, as indicated by the consistency of two very similarly done studies that were conducted about two decades apart (Farina and Ring 1965; Piner and Kahle 1984). The research has been summarized as follows: "Old and young, country and city dwellers, rich and poor, men and women, bright and dull, all regard people with mental disorders as fundamentally tainted and degraded" (Farina 1982). These feelings can be extremely strong. Thus, Gussow and Tracy (1968) had subjects evaluate various degrading conditions and reported that people believe the two most horrible things that can befall a person are leprosy and insanity. And when the attitudes toward these two maladies are compared, we find that, relative to the "leper," the "insane person" is regarded as more insecure, unpredictable, bad, tense, foolish, and dangerous (Nunnally 1961, pp. 270–272). Most people even believe that a mother would choose someone who has been convicted of a crime and jailed to care for her baby over someone who has been a mental patient (Lamy 1966). These unfavorable feelings on the part of the public are likely to make conditions in the community unpleasant for anyone toward whom they are directed. These feelings would seem to be especially destructive when the person subjected to them has recently been sufficiently maladjusted to require hospitalization and probably has a lot of self-doubts.

Evidence abounds that people with a history of mental disorder are treated in a disagreeable and hurtful way. This even happens within the confines of psychiatric hospitals, which are presumed to be havens for such individuals (Caudill et al. 1952; Rosenhan 1973). Once back in the community, if the individual is known to have been a psychiatric patient, a profusion of negative consequences are likely to be encountered by that individual even in the absence of any justification for these negative feelings in the appearance or behavior of the former patient. Carefully controlled laboratory experiments using male subjects show that others will want to avoid future contact with the former psychiatric patient, perceive in his behavior inadequacies that do not objectively exist, and inflict more pain upon him than they do upon control subjects (Farina and Ring 1965; Farina et al. 1966a). Studies done in the community make it clear that a history of mental disorder increases the problems of obtaining employment, finding lodgings, and perhaps even getting medical help (e.g., Farina and Felner 1973; Farina et al. 1976; Page 1977). And at least in the case of male former mental patients, if they do find a job, their extra problems are by no means over once their history becomes known to their coworkers (Farina et al. 1978).

The Impact of Social Stigma on the Stigmatized

Imagine an encounter between a man who has recently returned to his community after hospitalization for a mental disorder and an acquaintance who lives in the former patient's neighborhood. The latter knows about the hospitalization, and the former patient is aware that he knows. It seems intuitively obvious that the ensuing interaction will be tense and unpleasant. Part of the reason for these feelings was considered in the preceding section. That is, the "normal" member contributes to the difficulty by his stereotypic beliefs about mental patients. But the "normal" person is not the only member of the pair, and he may not be the only contributor to the ongoing interpersonal problems. It seems likely that the stigma is more important and salient to the afflicted than to the observer, and the blemished person's perceptions and comportment may be influenced by the stigma independently of how others behave. Research makes it clear that this is precisely what happens.

In one relevant study, male college students were asked to copy for transmission to another student either a history of a mental disorder or some bland information (Farina et al. 1968). In both conditions the subject was told that what was copied would be read by the other student. Actually, the information given to the other student was always the bland control statement regardless of what had been copied. In this way, only the belief of one of the students in each pair was varied. The results showed unambiguously that believing he was viewed as a former mental patient influenced the believer's behavior and, moreover, caused the other subject to reject him. Thus we see that social stigma influences the stigmatized person's behavior independently of how others act. The effect of this stigma seems to be such as to make the readjustment of deinstitutionalized patients more difficult. We see here a self-fulfilling prophecy. Because someone expects to be degraded and rejected, he actually causes the rejection he expects and fears.

However, it remained to be shown if real mental patients behave this way. For this reason, a second study was done on subjects who had been psychiatric patients at a VA hospital that also treats medical and surgical patients (Farina et al. 1971). They were asked to participate in a study that, allegedly, was to find out whether employers discriminate against former mental patients in their hiring practices. Hence, the subjects would meet one of a group of employment interviewers brought to the hospital to evaluate the potential of patients as workers. To determine if there was bias, some of the interviewers knew that the subjects were former psychiatric patients, while others were told that the subjects were former *medical* patients. Half the subjects were then informed that the interviewer knew they had been mental patients, while the rest were assured that the interviewer thought they had been medical patients. In fact, all subjects met the same confederate who was unaware of what they had been told and who made ratings of the former patients' behavior. All subjects were required to do a task, explain it to the "employment interviewer," and complete a questionnaire measuring their feelings and perceptions.

A very consistent and comprehensible pattern of results emerged. When the subjects believed the interviewer was aware of their status as former mental patients, they felt less appreciated, found the task more difficult, and performed more poorly than did those subjects in the control condition. Subjects in the mental patient condition were also rated by the "employment interviewer" as being more tense, anxious, and poorly adjusted than those in the control condition. Results highly consistent with those of the preceding study were reported by Link (1987), even though his procedures were very different. Together, these experiments indicate that both the feelings and the behaviors of former mental patients are adversely affected simply because these individuals think that other people know they have had a mental disorder. So we see that former mental patients face another difficulty fitting back into the community.

In addition to assessing the impact upon patients of believing that others are aware of their mental disorder, several other related issues have been investigated. One study compared the effect upon subjects of thinking they were definitely viewed as former mental patients with the effect of being uncertain if they were being viewed in such a way (Farina and Burns 1984). The results suggested that subjects in the former condition were more adversely affected than those in the latter. In several experiments, psychiatric patients were led to believe either that someone with whom they interacted had a favorable impression of patients like them and expected them to behave competently or else that the person with whom they interacted viewed patients as vulnerable, deviant, and incompetent (Luppino 1966; Rayne 1969; Thaw 1971). The results showed that patients are sensitive to the *specific* views that others have of them and respond in accordance with those views. In general, they perform better if they believe they are held in high regard and are viewed as being competent. This may happen because they are not motivated to do well when little is expected of them or possibly because they dare not confront the other person with an achievement of which the other considers them incapable.

Objective Characteristics of the Deinstitutionalized Population

Research has indicated that psychiatric patients possess characteristics that are widely devalued in our society. It may seem unkind to call attention to such aspects of people who are troubled emotionally and who already are socially degraded because of their difficulties in adjustment. However, these characteristics appear to be a barrier to their community readjustment, and we need to consider the role of these characteristics if we are to understand the process and help these individuals.

Societal and interpersonal incompetence. While the heterogeneity of psychiatric patients must be borne in mind, there is, nevertheless, one characteristic of mental patients that clearly differentiates them from the average person—that is, their relative lack of social relationships throughout their lives (Barthell and Holmes 1968; Farina and Webb 1956; Farina et al. 1962, 1963; Phillips 1953). Illustrative of these findings are the findings of Barthell and Holmes (1968), who examined the high school records of people who were later found to be normal, neurotic, or schizophrenic. They compared the three groups for number and type of activities in which they had engaged while in high school after classifying the activities as *social* or *nonsocial* in nature. An example of the former type of activity is membership in the student council, while an example of the latter is being a member of an athletic team. The authors found that the groups differed for social activities only, with the "normal" individuals having engaged in the most social activities, neurotic individuals having engaged in an intermediate amount, and schizophrenic individuals having engaged in the least amount. Another finding that was characteristic of research in this area was that the more severe the psychopathology an individual developed (i.e., schizophrenia vs. neurosis), the more sparse and fleeting were that person's interpersonal relationships prior to the onset of the disorder.

Given these histories, we would expect that, as a group, maladjusted individuals would not develop a rich repertoire of interpersonal behaviors nor understand social relationships and comport themselves skillfully with others. A great deal of research on various aspects of the interpersonal perception and behavior of people varying in adequacy of adjustment strongly and consistently supports these expectations. Thus, the findings of Farina et al. (1966b), who studied the social relationships of four groups of women differing in adequacy of adjustment, support the preceding expectations. From their findings Farina et al. concluded that the more poorly adjusted the subjects were, the more undifferentiated and amorphous were their perceptions of other people. For example, friends and enemies were much the same to them. Both Kelly et al. (1971) and Rosenthal (1973) have reported that among female patients, those whose adjustment was more adequate behaved more skillfully and appropriately in an interview with a stranger. Numerous other studies, done in a variety of ways and even in different countries, indicate that a chronic and quite general deficit in social competence is a prominent feature of maladjustment (Sarason and Sarason, 1987, p. 11). Walker et al. (1980) had schizophrenic and matched control subjects from three age groups identify emotions from photographs and found that the control subjects in each age group were better able to do this. Essentially the same study was done by Vandenberg (1962) and the same results were obtained. Turner (1964) had schizophrenic and control subjects listen to an actor convey six different emotions by means of a nonsense sentence. It was found that the schizophrenic subjects were less accurate than the control subjects in judging emotion when the voice, rather than the facial appearance, was used as a cue. These latter studies indicate that with increasing maladjustment, not only are people less able to display appropriate social behavior themselves, but also they are less competent to interpret the feelings being experienced by others, which would preclude their behaving in response to those feelings in ways that society expects.

As may be intuitively quite obvious, those individuals who do not behave in a socially appropriate manner are disliked and avoided. Greengrass (1974) used peer ratings to identify socially skilled and socially unskilled female college students and paired each of the subjects with a randomly assigned student. Each pair was required to discuss some problems for about 10 minutes. At the end of the discussion it was found that the socially competent subjects were liked better and were preferred as friends by the partners. Jain and Greengrass (unpublished manuscript, 1974) repeated this study and obtained the same results. Moreover, they found that the *partners* of the socially incompetent women were rated as being more uncomfortable during the interaction. Thus, the findings very likely indicate that it is stressful to socialize with interpersonally inept people. And in a longer-term study, Kelso (1978) measured how much students who rated high and low for social competence were liked by their peers at two points in time. Although after being together in a dormitory for 2 weeks there was no difference between the groups, by the end of the semester the subjects with high social competence were significantly better liked than the subjects with low social competence.

These patterns of interpersonal behaviors have been shown to be quite stable over time and appear to transcend episodes of acute psychiatric problems (Farina et al. 1957). The research thus suggests that deinstitutionalized psychiatric patients returning to the community behave in a socially inept fashion. It also implies that people in the community find these behaviors objectionable, which probably means that the former patients are rejected and, hence, find community readjustment difficult.

Alienating behaviors.   Another characteristic of psychiatric patients that distinguishes them from other men and women is symptoms of psychiatric disorders. Presumably it is the presence of these symptoms that is responsible for the classification of people as psychiatric patients and for their institutionalization. Psychiatric symptoms constitute a catalogue of behaviors that people evidently find noxious, disagreeable, or offensive and will avoid if possible. A very useful study of 793 patients admitted to a state psychiatric hospital (Zigler and Phillips 1961) provides us with information as to what these symptoms are and their frequency among psychiatric patients. Zigler and Phillips (1961) defined "symptom" as a characteristic of the patient as described by the admitting psychiatrist or a characteristic(s) that was listed by referring physicians as the reason for hospitalization. The nature of these symptoms and the percentage of patients manifesting these symptoms are shown in Table 15-1.

Abundant evidence exists clearly indicating that people who display the characteristic behaviors (or "symptoms") found in psychiatric patients (see Table 15-1) will be disliked and shunned. We will consider research pertinent to depression and tension, because they are the two most common of all psychiatric symptoms and they also may be the most fully investigated.

Coyne (1976), in what is probably the first study that bears on the issue of how the depressed patient is perceived, had college students interact over the telephone with depressed outpatients or with control subjects. Coyne found that relative to control subjects, depressed individuals were rejected and devalued, and moreover, the students who had talked with them were themselves depressed, anxious, and hostile after the conversation. Following Coyne's report, at least 11 additional similar studies were done (see Gurtman 1986 for a brief review).

It is apparent from a consideration of these studies that depressed people

Table 15-1. The most common symptoms displayed by a sample of psychiatric patients

Symptom	Percentage of patients ($N = 793$) displaying symptom
Depressed	38
Tense	37
Suspiciousness	35
Drinking	19
Hallucinations	19
Suicidal attempt	16
Suicidal ideas	15
Bodily complaints	15
Emotional outburst	14
Withdrawn	14
Perplexed	14
Assaultive	12
Self-deprecatory	12
Threatens assault	10
Sexual preoccupation	10

Source. Table adapted from Zigler and Phillips (1961).

are quite regularly rejected and that they arouse negative mood states in others, as Gurtman (1986) has concluded. Even studies quite differently done indicate that depressed individuals are particularly disagreeable to those around them. Coyne et al. (1987), in a later study, assessed individuals living with a depressed patient who was at the time experiencing a depressive episode. These individuals were compared with very similar subjects living with a depressed patient who was at the time *not* experiencing a depressive period. Coyne et al. found that the former subjects were very much more distressed than the latter. Particularly disturbing to these individuals were the patient's lack of interest in social life, fatigue, hopelessness, and worry. The findings of a study by Hooley et al. (1987) were very consistent with those of Coyne et al.'s. Hooley et al. found that wives of depressed psychiatric patients were more unhappy with their marriage than wives of nondepressed psychiatric patients with seemingly more obtrusive and florid symptoms. Thus, on the safe assumption that psychiatric hospitals cannot fully cure mental disorders, we can predict that a sizeable minority of deinstitutionalized patients will encounter negative social responses because they are depressed.

The harmful effect of tension on social relationships is even clearer. The most relevant information is provided by a series of five studies designed to reveal how acceptable as a co-worker an applicant who was tense and nervous would be to employees already on the job. (See Farina et al. 1978 for a summary of these studies.) Samples of employees met a candidate who was allegedly applying for the same job that they held. For half the subjects, the candidate behaved in a calm and relaxed manner, while for the remainder the candidate was tense and anxious. To appear tense, the candidate in all five studies displayed the following behavior: he or she seldom looked the employee in the eye, the head was kept down, the hands were sometimes wrung, and there was occasional swallowing as if his or her throat were dry. The experiment was done five times using five different candidates, and a new sample of employees was obtained for each replication. The employees who participated in the studies worked at three different places: a department store, a VA hospital, and the plant maintenance division of a state university.

The effect of tension, which was virtually identical across the five studies, was strong and unmistakable. Whether male or female, former mental patient or average person, the tense individual was uniequivocally rejected by both men and women. The consistency and strength of the findings are noteworthy in an area of research in which inconsistency is common. Of course, we should find out why society responds to tense people in this manner. But concerning our more practical goal of understanding the consequences of deinstitutionalization, these results speak eloquently. Those discharged psychiatric patients who are tense, rather than finding support and welcome, will meet antipathy and rejection in the community. It appears to us that this social reaction constitutes a major bar to eventual successful readjustment.

Physical attractiveness.   There are at least three published studies reporting that psychiatric patients are perceived as being less good looking than comparable control subjects (Archer and Cash 1985; Farina et al. 1977; Napoleon et al. 1980). The study by Napoleon et al. also provides evidence indicating that it is people's unattractiveness that causes them to have psychiatric problems rather than their maladjustment causing them to be unattractive. Despite the fact that Sussman and Mueser (1983) obtained negative results, the findings as a whole, particularly when relevant research with nonpsychiatric subjects is taken into account, suggest that poorly adjusted individuals are less good looking than those enjoying good mental health. Regarding nonpsychiatric subjects, at least 10 additional studies have looked for a comparable association between attractiveness and a variety of indices of adjustment for subjects who were not hospitalized psychiatric patients. Generally the subjects were college students. One of these studies (Noles et al. 1985) found no association between the two variables. But the other 9 report evidence indicating that the variables are related and that, as was the case for psychiatric inpatients, the less good looking the subjects, the more maladjusted they were likely to be (Barocas and Vance 1974; Burns and Farina 1987; Cash 1985; Cash and Begley 1976; Cash and Smith 1982; Mathes and Kahn 1975; O'Grady 1982, 1989; Umberson and Hughes 1987).

We certainly are not suggesting that any given psychiatric patient is less attractive than anyone who has not experienced psychiatric difficulties. We do not even believe that appearance is the major variable in the readjustment problems encountered by former psychiatric patients. However, if former psychiatric patients are relatively unattractive, then a great deal of research (e.g., Herman et al. 1986) makes it very clear that they will be treated more negatively than would otherwise be the case. This disagreeable and demeaning social reception, including rejection of their friendship and cruel treatment, will make readjustment to the community more difficult.

The research on attractiveness implies that the more unattractive deinstitutionalized psychiatric patients are, the less cordial will their social reception be and, hence, the more difficult their readjustment. This possibility was tested by Farina et al. (1986) with a group of psychiatric patients of both sexes who were about to be discharged to the community. The subjects' looks were rated at the time they were discharged. It was found that for both sexes, but more clearly for females, the better looking the patient was, the more successful he or she was in readjusting to community living. In addition to unattractiveness, more disturbed individuals are less likely to take care of themselves and consequently appear dirty and disheveled (Farina et al. 1957, Items 30 and 31). This inattention to appearance, perhaps more than inherent unattractiveness, seems likely to lead to community rejection.

Conclusion

We have systematically reviewed research on the social stigmatization of psychiatric patients. We undertook this effort hoping the research would provide a better understanding of the problems encountered in deinstitutionalizing patients and perhaps suggest ways to overcome those difficulties. The studies in the three areas reviewed (i.e., the social degradation of mental patients, the deleterious effect on the patients of this degradation, and the socially disliked characteristics of the patient population) show why psychiatric patients find it difficult to return to the community. Of course, some of what the research reveals has long been known to mental health workers. Indeed, programs have been established that are tailored specifically to reduce the problems that, as the research reviewed indicates, are faced by patients. Thus, McFall and his coworkers (e.g., Goldsmith and McFall 1975) have developed a system of teaching social skills to psychiatric patients that seems to be very effective, as the studies reviewed showing the lack of interpersonal skills of such individuals indicate it would be. However, careful attention to this research could increase our understanding and perhaps play a valuable heuristic role. The following example serves to illustrate this point.

A large number of studies have compared the effect of routine full-time hospitalization to alternative care (AC) procedures, particularly day care, but also home treatment and visits at home by public health nurses. The results consistently show that the effect of AC treatment is at least as good and typically better than that of traditional psychiatric hospital treatment. The most convincing studies have randomly assigned psychiatric patients to either hospitalization in a psychiatric institution or AC treatment. Kiesler and Sibulkin (1987) have recently reviewed 14 such studies and come to the same conclusions reached by previous reviewers. They illustrate these conclusions with the following quotation from an earlier review by Greene and De La Cruz (1981), whose conclusion specifically encompasses deinstitutionalization: "[A] review of the comparative studies on day treatment as an alternative modality to traditional full-time hospitalization reveals impressive evidence of its superior effectiveness in facilitating the adjustment and reintegration of patients into the community" (Greene and De La Cruz, p. 191). But if the patients are followed after treatment, the investigators find that the advantage of the AC group eventually disappears: "It seems quite clear from this array of studies that whatever differences exist between the AC and H [hospitalization] conditions after treatment dissipate over time" (Kiesler and Sibulkin 1987, p. 175).

Researchers have apparently not attempted to explain these findings. However, an explanation is possible if we recollect the first and second categories of studies reviewed. Society stigmatizes individuals who have adjustment problems; it differentiates such problems according to severity, and the more serious the disorder, the greater the social stigma engendered. Thus it seems very likely that the hospitalized individual is perceived as being more disordered than the one in alternative care and that the former will consequently be more unfavorably treated in the community. This in turn will make it more difficult to readjust. Also, the patients are aware of the more negative attitudes held toward hospitalized patients relative to patients in alternative care, and the hospitalized patients are correspondingly more adversely affected than those in alternative care conditions. Finally, it seems reasonable that the impact of the hospitalization, both on the former patient and on the community resident, would be greater immediately after discharge than later on when the emotional impact of the event would have had time to fade. And so we should expect to find that the difference between the hospitalized group and the AC group would become smaller with the passage of time.

Evidence does not exist to support all the elements of the foregoing explanation. However, research on social stigma does suggest the foregoing hypothesis, which could be tested with additional studies. We believe other findings in the general area of deinstitutionalization will be clarified by what research on stigma has revealed and continues to reveal.

References

Anthony WA, Buell GJ, Sharratt S, et al: Efficacy of psychiatric rehabilitation. Psychol Bull 78:447–456, 1972

Archer RP, Cash TF: Physical attractiveness and maladjustment among psychiatric patients. Journal of Social and Clinical Psychology 3:170–180, 1985

Barocas R, Vance FL: Physical appearance and personal adjustment counseling. Journal of Consulting Psychology 21:96–100, 1974

Barthell CN, Holmes DS: High school yearbooks: a non-reactive measure of social isolation in graduates who later became schizophrenic. J Abnorm Psychol 73:313–316, 1968

Burns GL, Farina A: Physical attractiveness and self-perception of mental disorder. J Abnorm Psychol 96:161–163, 1987

Cash TF: Physical appearance and mental health, in The Psychology of Cosmetic Treatments. Edited by Graham JA, Kligman A. New York, Praeger, 1985, pp 196–216

Cash TF, Begley PJ: Internal-external control, achievement orientation and physical attractiveness of college students. Psychol Rep 38:1205–1206, 1976

Cash TF, Smith E: Physical attractiveness and personality among American college students. J Psychol 11:183–191, 1982

Caudill W, Redlich FC, Gilmore HR, et al: Social structure and interaction processes on a psychiatric ward. Am J Orthopsychiatry 22:314–334, 1952

Coyne JC: Depression and the response of others. J Abnorm Psychol 85:186–193, 1976

Coyne JC, Kessler RC, Tal M, et al: Living with a depressed person. J Consult Clin Psychol 55:347–352, 1987

Farina A: Are women nicer people than men? Sex and the stigma of mental disorder. Clinical Psychology Review 1:223–243, 1981

Farina A: The stigma of mental disorders, in In the Eye of the Beholder. Edited by Miller AG. New York, Praeger, 1982, pp 305–363

Farina A, Burns GL: The effect of uncertainty as to whether others believe that one has had a mental disorder. Journal of Social and Clinical Psychology 2:244–257, 1984

Farina A, Felner RD: Employment interviewer reactions to former mental patients. J Abnorm Psychol 82:268–272, 1973

Farina A, Ring K: The influence of perceived mental illness on interpersonal relations. J Abnorm Psychol 70:47–51, 1965

Farina A, Webb WW: Premorbid adjustment and subsequent discharge. J Nerv Ment Dis 124:612–613, 1956

Farina A, Arenberg D, Guskin S: A scale for measuring minimal social behavior. Journal of Consulting Psychology 21:265–268, 1957

Farina A, Garmezy N, Zalusky N, et al: Premorbid behavior and prognosis in female schizophrenic patients. Journal of Consulting Psychology 26:56–60, 1962

Farina A, Garmezy N, Barry H: The relationship of marital status to incidence and prognosis of schizophrenia. Journal of Abnormal and Social Psychology 67:624–630, 1963

Farina A, Holland CH, Ring K: The role of stigma and set in interpersonal interaction. J Abnorm Psychol 71:421–428, 1966a

Farina A, Holtzberg J, Kimura DS: A study of the interpersonal relationships of female schizophrenic patients. J Nerv Ment Dis 142:441–444, 1966b

Farina A, Allen JG, Saul BB: The role of the stigmatized in affecting social relationships. J Pers 36:169–182, 1968

Farina A, Gliha D, Boudreau LA, et al: Mental illness and the impact of believing others know about it. J Abnorm Psychol 77:1–5, 1971

Farina A, Hagelauer HD, Holtzberg JD: Influence of psychiatric history on physicians' response to a new patient. J Consult Clin Psychol 44:499, 1976

Farina A, Fischer EH, Sherman S, et al: Physical attractiveness and mental illness. J Abnorm Psychol 86:510–517, 1977

Farina A, Murray PJ, Groh T: Sex and worker acceptance of a former mental patient. J Consult Clin Psychol 46:887–891, 1978

Farina A, Burns G, Austad C, et al: The role of physical attractiveness in the readjustment of discharged psychiatric patients. J Abnorm Psychol 95:139–143, 1986

Goldsmith JB, McFall RM: Development and evaluation of an interpersonal skill-training program for psychiatric inpatients. J Abnorm Psychol 84:51–58, 1975

Greene LR, De La Cruz A: Psychiatric day treatment as alternative to and transition from full-time hospitalization. Community Ment Health J 17:191–202, 1981

Greengrass MJ: Interpersonal behavior of people selected as socially skilled and unskilled. Unpublished master's thesis, University of Connecticut, Storrs, CT, 1974

Gurtman MB: Depression and the response of others: reevaluating the reevaluation. J Abnorm Psychol 95:99–101, 1986

Gussow Z, Tracy GS: Status, ideology, and adaptation to stigmatized illness: a study of leprosy. Human Organization 27:316–325, 1968

Herman CP, Zanna MP, Higgins ET (eds): Physical Appearance, Stigma, and Social Behavior: The Ontario Symposium, Vol 3. Hillsdale, NJ, Lawrence Erlbaum, 1986

Hooley JM, Richters JE, Weintraub S, et al: Psychopathology and marital distress: the positive side of positive symptoms. J Abnorm Psychol 96:27–33, 1987

Kelly FS, Farina A, Mosher DL: Ability of schizophrenic women to create a favorable or unfavorable impression on an interviewer. J Consult Clin Psychol 36:404–409, 1971

Kelso FW: The role of physical attractiveness and other variables in determining how much a person is initially and subsequently liked. Unpublished master's thesis, University of Connecticut, Storrs, CT, 1978

Kiesler CA, Sibulkin AE: Mental Hospitalization. Newbury Park, CA, Sage, 1987

Lamb HR, Goertzel V: The long-term patient in the era of community treatment. Arch Gen Psychiatry 34:679–682, 1977

Lamy RE: Social consequences of mental illness. J Consult Clin Psychol 30:450–454, 1966

Link BG: Understanding labeling effects in the area of mental disorders: an assessment of the effects of expectations of rejection. American Sociological Review 52:96 112, 1987

Luppino AV: The nature of chronic schizophrenia: implications derived from the effects of social reinforcement on performance. Unpublished doctoral dissertation, University of Connecticut, Storrs, CT, 1966

Mathes EW, Kahn A: Physical attractiveness, happiness, neuroticism, and self-esteem. Journal of Psychology 90:27–30, 1975

May CD: Resistance rises to group homes for mental cases. New York Times, March 24, 1986, B1, 4

Megan K: Hartford Courant, March 2, 1985, B1

Napoleon T, Chassin L, Young RD: A replication and extension of "physical attractiveness and mental illness." J Abnorm Psychol 89:250–253, 1980

Nickerson C: Reformer's dream that went astray. Boston Sunday Globe, March 10, 1985, pp 1, 22

Noles SW, Cash TF, Winstead BA: Body image, physical attractiveness and depression. J Consult Clin Psychol 53:88–94, 1985

Nunnally JC: Popular Conceptions of Mental Health. New York, Holt, Rinehart & Winston, 1961

O'Grady KE: Sex, physical attractiveness and perceived risk of mental illness. J Pers Soc Psychol 43:1064–1071, 1982

O'Grady KE: Physical attractiveness, need for approval, social self-esteem, and maladjustment. Journal of Social and Clinical Psychology 8:62–69, 1989

Page S: Effects of the mental illness label in attempts to obtain accommodation. Canadian Journal of Behavioral Science 9:84–90, 1977

Pepper B, Kirshner MC, Ryglewicz H: The young adult chronic patient: overview of a population. Hosp Community Psychiatry 32:463–469, 1981

Phillips L: Case history data and prognosis in schizophrenia. J Nerv Ment Dis 117:515–525, 1953

Piner KE, Kahle LR: Adapting to the stigmatizing label of mental illness: foregone but not forgotten. J Pers Soc Psychol 47:805–811, 1984

Rayne JT: The effect of perceived attitudes on expectancy for punishment by psychiatric patients. Unpublished doctoral dissertation, University of Connecticut, Storrs, CT, 1969

Rhinelander DH: Hartford Courant, May 20, 1983, B3

Rosenhan DL: On being sane in insane places. Science 179:250–258, 1973

Rosenthal BS: Schizophrenics' reactions to social roles as a function of social skills. Unpublished master's thesis, University of Connecticut, Storrs, CT, 1973

Sarason IG, Sarason BR: Abnormal Psychology. Englewood Cliffs, NJ, Prentice-Hall, 1987

Sussman S, Mueser KT: Age, socioeconomic status, severity of mental disorder, and chronicity as predictors of physical attractiveness. J Abnorm Psychol 92: 255–258, 1983

Thaw J: The reactions of schizophrenic patients to being patronized and to believing they are unfavorably viewed. Unpublished doctoral dissertation, University of Connecticut, Storrs, CT, 1971

Torrey EF: Hartford Courant, April 18, 1986, B11

Turner JB: Schizophrenics as judges of vocal expressions of emotional meaning, in The Communication of Emotional Meaning. Edited by Davitz JR. New York, McGraw-Hill, 1964

Umberson D, Hughes M: The impact of physical attractiveness on achievement and psychological well-being. Social Psychology Quarterly 50:227–236, 1987

Vandenberg SG: La mesure de la deterioration de la comprehension sociale dans la schizophrenie. Revue de Psychologie Appliquée 12:189–199, 1962

Walker E, Marwit SJ, Emory E: A cross-sectional study of emotion recognition in schizophenics. J Abnorm Psychol 89:428–436, 1980

Zigler E, Phillips L: Psychiatric diagnosis and symptomatology. Journal of Abnormal and Social Psychology 63:69–75, 1961

Chapter 16

The Psychiatric Hospital and Reduction of Stigma

Robert Gibson, M.D.

In this brief chapter the president of Sheppard-Pratt Hospital examines ways in which the psychiatric hospital can be an effective force in overcoming the stigma of mental illness. Dr. Gibson describes attempts at combating the invisibility that has often shrouded hospitals and patients. He also focuses on the development of a constituency as a powerful weapon to overcome the barriers created by stigma. Volunteer programs, collaboration with advocacy groups, and educational programs are key aspects in the development of such a constituency. Dr. Gibson urges hospitals to be proactive, to become part of the solution to the problem of stigma.

In this brief chapter the president of Sheppard-Pratt Hospital examines ways in which the psychiatric hospital can be an effective force in overcoming the stigma of mental illness. Dr. Gibson describes attempts at combating the invisibility that has often shrouded hospitals and patients. He also focuses on the development of a constituency as a powerful weapon to overcome the barriers created by stigma. Volunteer programs, collaboration with advocacy groups, and educational programs are key aspects in the development of such a constituency. Dr. Gibson urges hospitals to be proactive, to become part of the solution to the problem of stigma.

Stigma against mentally ill persons seems to have been present from the beginning of recorded history. Patients were held in prisons under the most deplorable conditions. Moses Sheppard, the founder of Sheppard-Pratt Hospital, was one of those who sought to achieve reform. A colleague of Moses Sheppard reported that Sheppard

> was horrified at the sight of the treatment extended to the insane paupers. . . . Men and women were crowded into narrow cells, stripped of every comfort, chained to the floor, or braced to the miserable apologies for beds and literally forced to wallow in filth. Custom had deadened the sensibilities of the public; a sufficient excuse for brutality. (Forbush 1968, pp. 202–203).

Sheppard's emphasis on "deadened sensibilities" highlights his concern about the impact of stigma.

In the late 1700s and early 1800s, several institutions were created to provide humane treatment and respite for mentally ill persons. For these pioneer institutions, the concept of asylum or treatment was a place to which the vulnerable could escape, be safe, and be protected from seizure or harm. Over the years, the term "asylum" changed, so that by 1961 Goffman used the title *Asylums* in his classic work to describe the demoralizing and disorganizing impact that institutions had when patients were sequestered and lacked adequate treatment.

Over time, asylum came to symbolize all that was fearsome about mental illness. Think of the origin of the word *bedlam*, which we use to mean disorganized, disrupted, and in disarray. It has its origin from the Hospital of St. Mary of Bethlehem in London; bedlam is a corruption of Bethlehem. Stigma thus became particularly associated with inpatient hospitalization.

The hospital or asylum became inextricably associated with mental illness itself; it became the symbol for all the frightening characteristics of the inmates of these hospitals, reinforcing the fear and adding to the stigma. The early mental hospitals were built in remote locations; usually surrounded by a fence or wall, these hospitals were fortress-like structures that emphasized security, with bars on windows and massive, indestructible oak furniture. Almost every problem was solved by increased security that was always additive and rarely withdrawn.

Little was done to change this situation until the decades of the 1950s and 1960s, when positive changes were initiated: hospitals moved toward an open-door policy; security screens, then unbreakable glass, were substituted for the bars; staff stopped wearing uniforms; and patients began to wear their own clothing. The community mental health center movement brought the treatment setting from isolated locations into the community. Despite all of these changes, mental hospitals continue to be the symbol of mental illness, with the associated negative aura and image.

In response to criticisms, psychiatric hospitals have developed a defensive reaction—that is, trying to avoid stigma by becoming invisible. I am especially sensitive to this, because I have lived on the grounds of Sheppard-Pratt for 25 years. For example, hospitals have used a box number for the return address on the hospital envelope. The reasoning was that if people received a letter from a psychiatric hospital that passed through the hands of a secretary or even the postman, it would tell the world that the recipients had some dealing with psychiatry and brand them with the stigma of mental illness.

The quest for invisibility has led hospitals to refuse to respond to inquiries about patients. Patients are "protected" from being photographed or interviewed even when they are willing to sign an authorization. A recent experience has led Sheppard-Pratt to reevaluate this policy. A news commentator of a local television station in Baltimore proposed a series about mental illness and hospital treatment programs. He made it clear at the outset that he wanted to have direct involvement with the patients so that they could appear in the program. Although several patients willingly signed clearances, many of our staff members thought it a dangerous practice that would be injurious to patients. Nevertheless, the interviews were permitted, forming the basis of four 8-minute segments in which some 10 patients appeared (broadcast in February 1989) ("State of Mind" 1989). The patients, who were named in the interviews, talked openly about their illnesses. As part of the program, the commentator carefully explained that the hospital protected confidentiality, but that these patients had asked to be identified in these extraordinarily moving interviews.

After the airing of the television programs, patients reported that the experience had been positive: family and friends had expressed pride in them, there was no negative feedback, and all reported feeling good about what they had done. Perhaps our benevolent paternalism has served more to perpetuate stigma rather than to protect the patients.

How can hospitals overcome the twin problems of indifference and stigma? A powerful weapon is development of a *constituency*, a term borrowed deliberately from the political arena to identify a group of supporters that provide a power base.

There are approaches that can be used to cultivate a constituency that will overcome the barriers created by stigma. Instead of being defensive, sequestered, withdrawn, and invisible, psychiatric hospitals should become a positive force and a part of the community. They should be proactive and break down barriers.

A volunteer program can be a powerful force in overcoming stigma. Volunteers are valuable in many ways: they provide substantial services; they bring diverse skills; and they raise money for patient services. It is equally important that each volunteer become an emissary representing the hospital in the community. When volunteers hear a distorted version of what goes on in a mental hospital, they can authoritatively say, "That isn't so. I am a volunteer at the hospital. I work with the patients. What you are saying is just not true." In short, volunteers are part of a strong, well-informed constituency.

Collaboration with advocacy and self-help groups offers another opportunity in the fight against stigma. In increasing numbers these groups include mental health associations, the National Alliance for the Mentally Ill, groups for depression and related affective disorders, Alcoholics Anonymous and its related groups, groups for anorexia and bulimia, and many more. There is much that professionals can learn from the positive and constructive accomplishments of these organizations. It is essential that the psychiatric hospital make a concerted effort to support the work of these organizations through such approaches as helping with their newsletters, providing meeting areas, and referring patients and their families for help.

Psychiatric hospitals have provided educational programs for mental health professionals over many years. These programs have seldom focused on the issue of stigma. They more often have been oriented toward the discussions of specific mental illnesses such as depression, schizophrenia, and Alzheimer's disease. While interested in disease-related topics, our audiences, in addition, want to learn about topical areas related to their own personal needs. For example, they want to know how to cope with anger, how to deal with difficult people, and how to improve family and couple relationships. The desire for information that will promote health seems to be almost endless.

The emphasis of educational programs is usually on overcoming ignorance through a didactic presentation. The impact is at the cognitive level through acquisition of knowledge. But overcoming stigma requires the changing of attitudes, not just the acquisition of skills or knowledge. Holding meetings at the hospital helps overcome the mystery. Using patients as tour guides dispels misconceptions. Exposure to patients who are functioning effectively helps break down stereotypes.

Mental illness is a serious, frightening disease. Much can be done to overcome ignorance and irrational fears that create stigma. And we must overcome stigma because it is one of the most serious barriers to treatment and to society's provision of the resources needed for adequate care of mentally ill persons.

Hospitals have become the symbol of mental illness because of the concentration of patients and the high visibility of the institution. As the symbol of mental illness, the hospital does send the message, "This is what mental illness is." The message may be distorted, but the perception is what counts. Trying to become invisible does not work. Isolation seems ominous and only adds to the mystery and fear of that place behind the walls.

We must be proactive. We must reach out. We must become highly visible. We must be highly articulate. We must develop a strong constituency if we are to overcome stigma. We need a constituency that understands not only the nature of mental illness but also the value of mental health promotion through human development and personal growth. Not until everyone is part of the constituency that is concerned about illness will we truly have overcome stigma.

Because hospitals are the symbol of mental illness, they are either part of the solution or part of the problem.

References

Forbush B: Moses Sheppard, Quaker Philanthropist of Baltimore. Philadelphia, PA, JB Lippincott, 1968

Goffman E: Asylums. New York, Doubleday, 1961

State of Mind, Parts 1–4. Television broadcast, WMAR TV, Baltimore, MD, Feb 1989

Chapter 17

The Stigma of Electroconvulsive Therapy: A Workshop

This chapter contains highlights from a workshop on electroconvulsive therapy (ECT) that was presented at the 1989 annual meeting of the American Psychiatric Association in San Francisco. ECT is a technically advanced and effective treatment that is often misunderstood and maligned by the lay public and by psychiatrists as well. Panel members probed the misinformation and myths that stigmatize this form of therapy. The psychosocial and semantic aspects of the problem were reviewed and suggestions offered to reduce stigma. For example, words like "shock," "seizure," and "convulsive" should be eliminated. The fear of ECT must be dispelled so that this therapy can be viewed correctly as a treatment of disease rather than as a punishment for social deviance.

The workshop participants point out that depressive disorders can be treated effectively with ECT. Yet the symptoms of depression are not well known by the general public. By publicizing the symptoms of major depressive disorder, the stigma of mental illness and of ECT as a treatment for a particular mental illness can be alleviated.

Introduction

Donald P. Hay, M.D.

The year 1988 was the 50th anniversary of the introduction of electroconvulsive therapy (ECT). Since 1938, when first introduced by Cerletti and Bini, ECT has had a tumultuous history. While there has apparently been

---

This chapter contains highlights from a workshop on electroconvulsive therapy that was presented at the 1989 annual meeting of the American Psychiatric Association in San Francisco. The participants were Norman S. Endler, Ph.D., F.R.S.C.; Donald P. Hay, M.D. (Chairperson); Mark J. Mills, M.D., J.D.; Glen Peterson, M.D.; and Herzl Spiro, M.D., Ph.D.

an awareness of the continued effectiveness of this treatment, the reaction has been quite overwhelming and at times fraught with controversy. From 1938 to the 1950s, we saw an extensive use of ECT. During that period of time, ECT was the major treatment, if not frequently the only biological treatment, for mental illness.

From the 1950s through the 1970s, with the advent of psychotropic medications (including the development of neuroleptics and of tricyclic antidepressants), we saw a decline in the use of ECT. In the 1970s, concern developed regarding the side effects of psychotropic medications, including the cardiovascular effects of the tricyclic antidepressants and the potential for tardive dyskinesia with neuroleptics. This concern resulted in a resurgence of interest in ECT and led to many studies and reports evaluating the effectiveness of this modality.

At the same time, the myths, misinformation, and public outcry continued. Senator Eagleton lost his vice-presidential bid when he revealed that he had received ECT. In the movie *One Flew Over the Cuckoo's Nest* (from Ken Kesey's novel), Jack Nicholson portrayed a patient receiving ECT for the wrong purpose (coercion) and in the wrong fashion (without anesthetic or muscle relaxant). In *Frances*, the movie about the actress Frances Farmer, a similar misrepresentation of ECT was shown. In both of these movies the ECT treatment was depicted as being followed by lobotomy, which reinforced the myth of ECT as a primitive, punitive procedure. Even in the critically acclaimed film *Ordinary People*, which exhibited an empathetic and intelligent portrayal of the role of psychiatry, ECT was maligned.

The "Berkeley Ballot," by which administration of ECT was outlawed in California for a period of time, exemplified issues of the ability or inability to provide a medical treatment in a particular part of the country by virtue of a public referendum. There are continuing restrictions of the ability to provide ECT in California, as in the case of *Doe v. O'Conner*.

While public concern continues as a result of negative media portrayal, progress in ECT has continued with significant medical advancements. "Modified" ECT, which includes the use of anesthesia, muscle relaxation, and improved ECT devices with pulsed square-wave apparatuses, has been developed.

In 1978 the American Psychiatric Association (APA) Task Force released a report on ECT that summarized information current to that time. The most recent APA Task Force on ECT, chaired by Richard D. Weiner, M.D., Ph.D., has been approved [published by the APA in 1990 as *The Practice of Electroconvulsive Therapy: Recommendations for Treatment, Training, and Privileging*]. The National Institutes of Health has addressed ECT issues in a Consensus Conference. There have been many studies and reports, and an entire journal, *Convulsive Therapy*, is devoted to ECT case reports and research.

In an effort to promote a better understanding of the paradox of a techni-cally advanced and effective treatment that is continually misunderstood and maligned, a workshop was presented at the 1989 APA annual meeting in San Francisco, California. The panel addressed various aspects of the stigma of ECT, including psychiatrists' attitudes, the social and political aspects, the psychosocial and semantic aspects, the legal aspects, and rec-ommendations for the future of ECT.

The following is a summary of some of the workshop proceedings.

Psychiatrists' Attitudes

Glen Peterson, M.D.

Even with the current state of advancement of other types of treatments in psychiatry, ECT is a uniquely important and sometimes life-saving treat-ment. Yet there is a relative trend among individuals and in different parts of the country to underutilize ECT.

Education has a very significant impact on psychiatrists' attitudes to-ward ECT. Some training programs offer no practical training in ECT, and their graduates may not even witness the treatment. In one survey of the members of the Association for Convulsive Therapy (ACT) that covered about 26 states, about 40% of the respondents said that their regional training programs did not provide training in ECT. A more formal compre-hensive survey is being completed at the University of Oregon. Both the American Board of Psychiatry and Neurology and the Residency Review Committee of the American Medical Association are aware of this situation. The American Psychiatric Association Task Force continues to address ECT issues.[1]

Psychiatrists in training who do not have much exposure to ECT are more likely to view it as a dangerous treatment. They are also less likely to develop an emotional, intuitive feeling to the specific conditions and at what phase of an illness ECT might be appropriate. Timeliness is of significant concern. Using ECT as a last resort seems to be one common approach. In many training programs psychotherapy and drugs are idealized and the impression of "unmodified" ECT evokes a negative image.

Subtle inhibitions against ECT exist in some communities. There is also the myth that there are few practitioners and facilities providing ECT, making it a low-profile treatment.

---

[1] See American Psychiatric Association Task Force: *The Practice of Electroconvul-sive Therapy: Recommendations for Treatment, Training, and Privileging.* Wash-ington, DC, APA, 1990.

Social and Political Aspects

Norman S. Endler, Ph.D., F.R.S.C.

One of the major goals of mental health workers should be to educate both the general public and those whom they train. Nevertheless, because of a sense of mystique and secretiveness, mental health workers may at times inadvertently further contribute to the stigma regarding mental illness (Endler and Persad 1988). A poignant example is the subject of depression and ECT. Many social workers and psychologists have negative attitudes towards ECT, mostly based on misinformation and myths. Most psychiatrists state that if they themselves were severely depressed, they would want ECT as the treatment of choice for them (Endler 1990; Endler and Persad 1988). The data indicate that ECT alleviates the symptoms for bipolar depression in 85% to 90% of all cases, as compared with antidepressants, with which the success rate is 65% to 70%.

Nevertheless, when a biological treatment is indicated, ECT is rarely the treatment of first choice. There are a number of "nonscientific" reasons for this state of affairs: 1) antidepressant drugs are less expensive; 2) it is easier and less time consuming to prescribe drugs; 3) ECT (even on an outpatient basis) necessitates a psychiatrist, a nurse, an anesthetist, equipment, a treatment room, and written consent; and 4) psychiatrists' concern and "worry" about the negative attitudes of the public toward ECT create a reluctance to prescribe it. Psychiatrists try antidepressant drugs as the treatment of first choice; if this approach does not work, then they may use ECT. We believe there is also an additional reason. Nobody, including psychiatrists, likes the idea of electricity applied to the brain. It is frightening, and furthermore the brain is considered the essence of the self—the core of "being." Consequently, as Endler and Persad (1988, p. 108) point out, "a depressed person who receives ECT may be doubly stigmatized; once for being mentally ill and then again for having undergone ECT . . ."

Psychosocial and Semantic Aspects

Herzl Spiro, M.D., Ph.D.

Public attitudes toward a procedure are shaped by several psychosocial and semantic factors. Maximum stigma will be attached to a procedure used as a punishment for willful social deviance. What if surgery were seen as the use of scalpels to cause pain, bleeding, and dismemberment for social deviants who willfully avoided work and family obligations? Suppose the layman's view of surgery was shaped by movies showing operations done without benefit of anesthesia to punish heroic rebels fighting an unfair surgery ward! The public then might well manifest prejudice against surgery.

The semantics of the term "electroconvulsive therapy," the confusion perpetrated by statements that mental illness is mythic, and the vivid portrayals of ECT in films such as *One Flew Over the Cuckoo's Nest* all contribute to such stigmatization. What shapes this stigma? We have considered elsewhere in some detail the issues of social deviance, sick roles, and stigmatization of mental illness (see Crocetti et al. 1974) and here briefly summarize our main conclusions.

ECT Viewed as the Consequence of Social Deviance Instead of as a Treatment for Disease

The attribution of cause determines whether one sees something as disease or social deviance. Social deviance is punished not only to deter the behavior but also to assert group cohesion (Durkheim 1933). When the perceived cause is the presence of medically defined disease, the "sick role" is permitted (Parsons 1958). As long as psychiatric disorders are seen as willful behaviors rather than as diseases, they will be perceived as being products of social deviance.

In addition to social attributions of causation, perceptions of the course of a disorder shape the social roles ascribed to individuals with that disorder. Many psychiatric disorders have a chronic course that does not fit the acute sick role. Chronic disease, in fact, tends to be placed into a different subgrouping—what Gordon (1966) has termed "the impaired role." The tendency to deny the sick role to those individuals with psychiatric illness contributes to viewing ECT as punishment. Social deviance is not treated, it is punished.

The key factor in attitude formation is the tendency one has to feel empathy for a person suffering from a given disorder. An individual who observes an abhorrent behavior might react with the thought, "There but for the grace of God go I." One can then ascribe a role that permits treatment. If one reacts with a feeling that this could never happen to oneself, then at that point there is a tendency to ascribe approaches that are more on the punitive side (Crocetti et al. 1974).

The nature of the treatment is another factor in determining attitudes. If someone is punished, the first assumption is that the person has done something that is punishable. Our studies revealed that people who were well acquainted with a backward state hospital system in the early 1970s had more negative attitudes toward mental illness than did people who did not visit the hospitals at all. In contrast, persons who visited a community mental health center with a very modern approach and respect for patient dignity had more positive attitudes the more they were exposed to that treatment method. When one sees a positive treatment in a medical setting, one is more inclined to ascribe a sick role to the person instead of attributing the behavior to social deviance.

Perceived locus of control also helps social attitudes. Any time the treatment of a condition involves vesting control in some remote authoritarian system, one is more likely to encounter negative attitudes. Administration of treatment to people coerced and held against their will inevitably will be seen as punishment.

Attitudes toward the treatment are affected by negative attitudes toward the disease being treated. Depressed individuals lack sufficient energy to work and perform daily tasks. This lack of energy can be attributed to laziness or it can be attributed to an imbalance of neurotransmitters in the brain. Depressed individuals cannot concentrate and therefore make many mistakes. This can be ascribed to either carelessness or sickness. Individuals who are depressed fail to respond to interpersonal cues and may frown or appear sad at times when other social responses would be more appropriate. Negative motives may consequently be attributed to the depressed person. The question is whether depression will be seen within a disease model or will be seen as an example of "self-indulgent, crying, lazy people who just will not do their work." Such conditions can readily be misinterpreted as social deviance, not deserving of sympathy and care. Thus, the tendency to see mental illness as social deviance rather than as a medical disorder results in its treatment being viewed in itself as a stigmatizing punishment.

Stigmatization of the Treatment

The second major factor in stigma formation is the nature of the treatment itself. The semantic issues become paramount. Modern ECT administered under anesthesia induces far less discomfort and medical sequelae than most surgical or pharmacological interventions. In this light, it is very inappropriate to call such treatment "shock therapy." Max Fink (1979) has pointed out that "shock" has a specific meaning: it is the perception of the passage of an electric current. This produces pain and discomfort. The word "shock" denotes perceptions that do not occur under anesthesia. This would be analogous to labeling surgery "pain therapy." Little wonder such a term as shock therapy engenders stigma.

The inappropriate use of language forms negative attitudes and prejudice. The words "convulsion" and "seizure" both have special meanings to the public. In studies of perceived social distance from different medical disorders, we have found that "convulsions" and "epilepsy" rank with "schizophrenia" in terms of negative attitudes. The mystification of convulsions goes back to ancient history when epilepsy and seizure disorders were seen as the disease of the gods—disorders that some spirit had inflicted on a person. It is not necessary to invoke all the prejudice and stigma of epilepsy and convulsive disorders to characterize the medical treatment of depression. Convulsions in the sense that laymen think of the term do not occur with modern ECT methods. "Seizure" is used in its technical sense to refer to the patterned electrical response produced by an electrical stimulus. However, that is not what the layperson thinks of when the word seizure is used. Why not use plain English and simply call the response what it is, "a patterned response," rather than using the term "seizure."

Semantic/Psychosocial Aspects of Stigma Reduction

Public education about the medical nature of depressive disorders will in the long run indirectly reduce the stigma attached to treatment methods such as ECT. The treatment itself should be given a new name that describes what is done in neutral, "unloaded" language. Words like "shock," "seizure," and "convulsive" should be eliminated. One proposed term is "cerebroversion," analogous to the term used in cardiology, "cardioversion." "Central stimulation" is another potential name for what we now call ECT. A more precise term would be "central stimulation with patterned response" (CSPR). "Brain stimulation therapy" (BST) would be equally neutral.

A clean break with the past is in order. Paying attention to semantic issues and the psychosocial origins of prejudice may make this procedure available to many more patients who need it.

Legal Aspects

Mark J. Mills, M.D., J.D.

Stigma is a relatively novel topic in that it is usual for patients to be stigmatized but, perhaps, not our own therapeutic modalities or the physician himself or herself. To some extent what happens with ECT is, if you will, a growth experience. It can be humbling; it can be informative; it can be consciousness raising. In terms of the legal issues involved there are four key topics: 1) what the law is, 2) the history of ECT, 3) what the anti-ECT laws have done, and 4) the law and the stigmatization of ECT.

What Is the Law?

The law is codified social policy and is any kind of societal interactive process. The law can be effected based on societal perceptions and, of course, on misperceptions. Unfortunately, as has been previously discussed, the movie *One Flew Over the Cuckoo's Nest* galvanized a great deal of not only public concern, but public outrage. Literally millions of viewers saw a repressive society brutalizing a compassionate individual or a creative individual in a way that was extraordinarily unbecoming. During that same period there was another movie, *Cool Hand Luke*, in which again an outspoken and courageous individual was repressed and brutalized by society. So, the laws that have regulated ECT reflect that kind of social perception and that kind of social misperception.

On the other hand, it is helpful to think of social policy and legal regulation as not occurring in a vacuum. It occurs in context, and the era during which the early anti-ECT laws were passed was when other things were occurring, some of which were frankly coercive and useful in society. This was a period of increasing regulation of civil commitment; by and large, the changed civil commitment laws required civil commitment to be much briefer and much more specific. There had to be a basis for civil commitment. That legislation probably has been a useful reform. Additionally, there were new concerns about informed consent. Most of those concerns have been useful. Taken for granted today, the process of getting an informed consent release prior to any kind of intrusive therapeutic process, whether it be pharmacological or surgical, is largely sensible. Additionally, this was the time of legislative activism, and in some cases, of course, of legislative optimism such as "The Great Society."

Electroconvulsive therapy was developed in 1938, well before the period of antipsychotic or neuroleptic medication and during the period in which there was relatively little hope in the treatment of schizophrenia or of serious affective disorders. This was the era of phenobarbital, or wet sheet packs, and of not very much else. It was an era in which kindness and compassion clearly made a difference, but in which there were very few meaningful treatments in our therapeutic armamentarium. It was also an era, of course, before the advent of histofluorescents and, therefore, before the advent of an understanding of neurotransmitters and neuropsychiatry, and the development of the catecholamine hypotheses of depression and schizophrenia.

It is still true, however, that the mechanisms for ECT remain only incompletely elucidated and that, although there are theories of increased membrane permeability, the mechanism of ECT is not adequately understood, even today. Nevertheless, medicine is very largely an empirical profession, and very often emphasis is not placed on how things work. There is concern that they do work, and this applies to something as simple as an aspirin tablet, the mechanism of which is still not totally understood even today.

It is clear that ECT frequently is remarkably ameliorative. Approximately 85% to 95% of people who have the indications for ECT, including serious depression and depression with delusions, respond rapidly and favorably. This is a level of therapeutic efficacy largely unknown elsewhere in medicine.

Finally, in the history of ECT use there have been abuses. Some patients, as described by George Winokur, have received over 500 ECT treatments. There were "shock shops" in the United States where physicians appeared to benefit, largely remuneratively, from providing this treatment. A study of ECT in Massachusetts published some time ago concluded that in the private sector, ECT appeared to be overutilized, at least in certain locales, but that it was underutilized in the public sector. The public sector had virtually abandoned ECT. For the delusionally depressed patient who could not afford to get a private physician, ECT was largely unavailable.

What the Anti-ECT Laws Have Done

The laws themselves have affected ECT. At the extreme, they have banned it outright, as of course occurred in the "Berkeley Ballot" several years ago. That referendum was ultimately set aside as an unwanted intrusion into an arena that questioned the degree of social intrusiveness reasonable for depressed patients and for those being treated with ECT.

The Law and Stigmatization of ECT

Two analogies can be used that probe various aspects of this legislation. The condition of low-pressure or normal-pressure hydrocephalus creates a condition in which one loses his or her capacity to do a number of things. Patients with this condition have gait apraxias and dementias that are potentially reversible. They are treated routinely with brain shunts placed in the central nervous system, largely rather successfully. This procedure does carry certain risk of morbidity, largely due to infections, and an occasional mortality. What is intriguing is that there is no law requiring that people who have low-pressure or normal-pressure hydrocephalus have somebody provide informed consent; have an external review, or have an external physician ratify their capacity to make an informed consent decision; or have an external reviewer (at least until the days of HMOs or other health care plans requiring external reviewers) to say that the surgical intervention is appropriate. In this procedure—one in which everyone who undergoes it is in effect incompetent—there is no social intrusiveness. This is due to the numbers alone. The people who have normal-pressure hydrocephalus are relatively few. One could also speculate that there has been no R. P. McMurphy (the character played by Jack Nicholson in *Cuckoo's Nest*) suffering from normal-pressure hydrocephalus coming under the knife.

Another analogy is cardiac bypass surgery, particularly in those patients who have postmyocardial infarction. This is a condition that, of course, has a period of known genuine and great peril, but at the same time there is no presumptive sense that persons who have had myocardial infarctions are in any way cognitively diminished. Common sense, however, dictates that when any of us are about to "meet our maker," we are naturally afraid or frightened and that most people in such a context will make decisions partly in a regressed state.

Again, the law does not say that individuals who suffer a serious myocardial infarction and are about to have bypass surgery must have that process validated by an external physician. Most would object to an outside physician coming in to ratify our capacity to give consent or to make recommendations to the surgeon planning to do the bypass surgery. This is due to the fact that the law views the psychiatric patient quite ambivalently. On the one hand, the trend of the law over the last several decades has been to presume competence. On the other hand, it is virtually indisputable that, irrespective of the law, the actual judges and courts that make the law perceive psychiatric patients as being somewhat different. Now, of course, for seriously ill patients, particularly schizophrenic individuals, this may be true. There are several elegant studies that suggest that those people who have schizophrenia, because their illness intrudes into their thought processes, remember less about their informed consent they made for ECT than would otherwise be predicted.

Undoubtedly some people with depression also encounter the same informed consent problem. However, the law has been unusually vigorous in the case of persons with depression, and to a very significant extent this reflects the kind of socially perceived problems that ECT has without a comparable understanding of the social benefits of ECT.

In combining all of these issues, a sense of meaning emerges in the relationship of the law and ECT. The combined effect is that stigma on the one hand and regulation on the other, largely at the state level, have meant a decreased use of one of the more successful psychotherapeutic alternatives (i.e., ECT) and, therefore, a decreased ability on the part of clinician and patients to make a rational decision about therapy.

Recommendations for the Future

Donald P. Hay, M.D.

It is evident that the treatment of ECT is efficacious and has relatively few side effects. The history and nature of this treatment, however, have left it with a legacy of negative image and underutilization. What can the psychiatric community do to overcome or improve this situation? One way is through education and dissemination of correct information.

It is important to convey that a series of biological diseases may occur in the brain for which there are biological treatments, including ECT. It is also important to explain that when an individual is biologically depressed, the same organ (the brain) that is ill may be dysfunctional to the point that the individual will not perceive (mind) that he or she needs treatment. A person with diabetes in which the mind is unaffected may more easily bring himself or herself to treatment than the biologically depressed in which the organ that is ill is the one that is used to make the decision of whether or not to go for help.

It is possible that individuals who become outraged at the prospect of treatments such as ECT may have confused true mental illness with the distress of the "worried well." Following this paradigm, psychiatrists are easily viewed as spending much of their time involuntarily hospitalizing individuals, prescribing so-called "mind-altering drugs," and providing ECT for behavior inconsistent with the psychiatrist's wishes and expectations. Remove the biological basis of emotional illness and it is easy to understand those who have been horrified of psychiatrists and their practices (Hay 1988).

The disease for which ECT is most effective is just as misunderstood as the treatment itself. Depression is a generic term that has many different meanings in our culture. It is important to distinguish, therefore, between the situational sadness that is understood by most individuals and the medical disease "depression" that is so effectively treated with ECT. In effect, it is easy to misinterpret the treatment as being punitive or manipulative if the disease is viewed as merely a sad mood due to situational events. As the knowledge increases regarding the biochemical etiology of depression, it becomes clearly appropriate to treat this illness with a medical procedure.

The symptoms of depressive disorder are well known in psychiatry, but are not well known by the general public. In the same way that the "8 warning signs of cancer" are well publicized by the media and relatively well known by the population, it would be helpful if the symptoms of major depressive disorder were easily identifiable and remembered. To this end a two-word mnemonic has been developed to help with this task: CEASE SAD. The letters of the two words spell out the 8 important symptoms of major depressive disorder as follows (Hay 1989):

Concentration decrease
Energy decrease
Anxiety increase
Spontaneous crying
Early morning wakening or other insomnia

Suicidal ideation
Appetite decrease or change
Deprecatory thoughts of self; guilt feelings

By using mnemonics such as CEASE SAD and other written and verbal forms of communication, education of the public is the most effective way of combating stigma, especially with regard to ECT.

There are many vehicles for promoting this knowledge. These include presentations at public lectures, appearances on radio and television shows, and articles in local newspapers, magazines, and newsletters. There are several textbooks on ECT and an extensive literature of research and studies (Abrams 1988; Abrams and Essman 1978; Fink 1979). Translation of this information by practitioners into understandable language for the general population is the best response to myth, misrepresentation, and stigma (Hay 1989, 1990a, 1990b; Hay and Hay 1990).

Adequate information when conveyed to the public will go a long way toward dispelling the fear that ECT is administered to control poor unfortunates and "shock" them into submission. We need to demystify who we are and what we do, the patients whom we treat, and the illnesses that beset them.

The cure for stigma is education. The resources are available. The responsibility is ours.

References

Abrams R: Electroconvulsive Therapy. New York, Oxford University Press, 1988

Abrams R, Essman WB: Electroconvulsive Therapy: Biological Foundations and Clinical Applications. New York, Spectrum, 1978

American Psychiatric Association: Electroconvulsive Therapy (APA Task Force Report No 14). Washington, DC, American Psychiatric Association, 1978

American Psychiatric Association: The Practice of Electroconvulsive Therapy: Recommendations for Treatment, Training, and Privileging (APA Task Force Report). Washington, DC, American Psychiatric Association, 1990

Crocetti GM, Spiro HR, Siassi I: Contemporary Attitudes Towards Mental Illness. Pittsburgh, PA, University of Pittsburgh Press, 1974

Endler NS: Holiday of Darkness, Revised Edition. Toronto, Wall & Thompson, 1990

Endler NS, Persad E: Electroconvulsive Therapy: The Myths and the Realities. Toronto, Hans Hubers Publishers, 1988

Fink M: Convulsive Therapy: Theory and Practice. New York, Raven, 1979

Freeman MB, Cheshire BA: Attitude studies on electroconvulsive therapy. Convulsive Therapy 2:31-42, 1986

Gordon GA: Role Theory and Illness: A Sociologic Perspective. New Haven, CT, Yale University Press, 1966

Hay DP: Treating depression: strategies for the brain and insights for the mind. Suicide Prevention Link, Wisconsin Chapter of the National Committee on Youth Suicide Prevention, Vol 3, No 4 (Winter), 1988

Hay DP: Electroconvulsive therapy in the medically ill elderly. Convulsive Therapy 5:8-16, 1989

Hay DP: ECT: safe and effective treatment for elderly psychiatric patients. Psychiatric Times, Nov 1990a, pp 49-50

Hay DP: Electroconvulsive therapy, mental health and aging. International Journal of Technology and Aging, Vol 3, 1990b, pp 39-45

Hay DP, Hay LK: The role of ECT in the treatment of depression, in Depression: New Directions in Research, Theory and Practice. Edited by Endler N. Toronto, Wall & Emerson, 1990, pp 255-272

Further Reading

Baxter LR, Roy-Byrne P, Liston EH, et al: Informing patients about electroconvulsive therapy: effects of a videotape presentation. Convulsive Therapy 2:25–29, 1986

Guze BH, Baxter LR, Liston EH, et al: Attorneys' perceptions of electroconvulsive therapy: impact of instruction with an ECT videotape demonstration. Compr Psychiatry 29:520–522, 1988

Hay DP: Malpractice insurance and consent regulations: Wisconsin experience. Convulsive Therapy 4:311–312, 1987

Hay DP: Electroconvulsive therapy, in Comprehensive Review of Geriatric Psychiatry. Edited by Sadavoy J, Lazarus LW, Jarvik LF. Washington, DC, American Psychiatric Press, 1991, pp 469–485

Hay DP, Hay LK, Spiro HR: The enigma of the stigma of ECT: 50 years of myth and misrepresentation. Wis Med J 88(12):4–8, 1989

Hughes J, Barraclough BM, Reeve W: Are patients shocked by ECT? J R Soc Med 74:283–287, 1981

Kramer BA: Use of ECT in California, 1977–1983. Am J Psychiatry 142:1190–1192, 1985

Parsons T: Definitions of health and illness in the light of American values and social structures, in Patients, Physicians, and Illness. Edited by Jaco WC. Glencoe, IL, Free Press, 1958, pp 165–187

Slawson P: Psychiatric malpractice: the electroconvulsive therapy experience. Convulsive Therapy 1:195–203, 1985

Chapter 18

The Stigmatization of Psychiatrists Who Work With Chronically Mentally Ill Persons

Howard Dichter, M.D.

In this chapter, Dr. Dichter summarizes key issues developed in earlier chapters. He examines the realities and myths surrounding the image of institutions, deinstitutionalization, electroconvulsive therapy, and social stereotyping of psychiatrists and formulates a five-component interactive model that highlights the major sources of stigma of psychiatrists who work with chronically mentally ill persons. He shows how the interaction of components multiplies the impact of stigma.

Dr. Dichter then determines specific activities that will reduce stigma. He argues for redefining the role of the psychiatrist to include leadership and administration in the treatment of chronically mentally ill persons. An expanded role for psychiatrists will result in both reduced stigma for the psychiatrist and better care for patients. Other suggestions include lobbying for funds, affiliating with universities, increasing the scope of residency training, and working with patient and family advocates. Together these activities comprise a forceful attack on stigma.

P sychiatrists who treat chronically mentally ill persons are "marked" by other psychiatrists, by other mental health workers, and by the mentally ill persons themselves and their families. The stereotype of the psychiatrist who works with this population is an unsuccessful (financially), over-worked psychiatrist who is considered to be incompetent or at least ineffective.

This stigma has been attributed to many causes. One explanation is that the stigma associated with these patients is "contagious"—that is, it is generalized from the chronically mentally ill patient to the treating psychiatrist. Other explanations, including low pay, ineffectiveness in "curing" patients, and cumbersome treatment systems, address more practical aspects of the psychiatrist's role within the general medical community (Talbott 1988). In this chapter I will discuss a five-component interactive model that highlights the major sources of stigma of psychiatrists who work with patients who are chronically mentally ill. More importantly, I will suggest activities that impact on this model to reduce the stigma of the psychiatrist treating chronically mentally ill persons. Decreasing or dissipating the stigma will lead to increased effectiveness and efficient use of the psychiatrist's unique role in treating this difficult population.

Sources of Stigma

The five major sources of stigma are patient stigma, the image of the psychiatrist, perceptions of past treatments, the current treatment system, and the economics of care. These sources and their impact on stigma are described below.

Patient Stigma

It is clear that the chronically mentally ill patient is stigmatized or "marked" by society. The stereotype of such a patient includes several critical elements that are usually associated with stigma, such as dangerousness and disruptive behavior, the patient's responsibility for his or her current condition ("Why doesn't this person just take a bath and clean up his act?"), unaesthetic appearance, and expectations of decline in functioning (Jones et al. 1984). Patient stigma is increased with the state of current service delivery, which has led to an increased number of mentally ill patients among the homeless. Patients living on the streets are more visible and often appear unaesthetic, disruptive, and dangerous. In addition, the expectation of long-term treatment from the community increases the stigma. The more chronically dependent that "marked" people become, the more intolerant others are of them (Jones et al. 1984).

The patient's stigma is transferred to the psychiatrist in two ways. First, the psychiatrist is stigmatized because he or she has chosen to work with the most stigmatized patients. Some assume anyone who wants to work with such a low-status patient group must lack initiative, training, and ambition. Second, when the patient displays asocial and/or dangerous behavior, the psychiatrist is thought to have failed to help the patient, "cure" the illness, or protect society from the mentally ill person. Fear and discomfort associated with the patient are generalized to the psychiatrist.

The Image of the Psychiatrist

There are a number of stereotypes of general psychiatrists (e.g., "crazy," mentally disturbed, sexually preoccupied, and aloof and distant). Two stereotypes especially directed toward those treating persons who are chronically mentally ill are the psychiatrist as drug pusher and the incompetent psychiatrist.

The "drug pusher" stereotype is reinforced by recent changes in the conceptualization of mental illness. Specifically, the remedicalization of psychiatry and the development of neurobiological explanations for major mental illness have increased the orientation toward pharmacological treatment of major mental illness. These paradigms, in conjunction with limited psychiatric resources in the community mental health centers, can narrow the psychiatrist's role to prescription writing. In the extreme case, psychiatrists are expected to see patients only when medication is indicated and for short periods of time (i.e., 30 minutes for an evaluation and 5–15 minutes for follow-up). In some settings, psychiatrists may be expected to sign blank prescriptions to be completed by nonmedical staff (a practice I find unethical).

Some patient advocates believe that prescribed medications are harmful. This belief has resulted from tendencies toward using medications to control agitation and anxiety in chronically mentally ill persons (Talbott 1988). The medications can exacerbate symptoms, especially flattened affect, withdrawal, and impoverished thinking (i.e., the negative symptoms of schizophrenia) (Andreasen 1984). Some medications can create new, irreversible symptoms, such as tardive dyskinesia, that can increase social stigma.

The second stereotype, the incompetent psychiatrist, is portrayed in the cinema. Psychiatrists are represented as eccentric buffoons insensitive to the patient's trauma, and incompetent, as in the movies *Nuts* and *Hairspray*. Psychiatrists may also be portrayed as vindictive. In the movies *Frances* and *One Flew Over the Cuckoo's Nest*, insulin shock and lobotomy were used to punish patients who evoked powerful negative feelings in psychiatrists and their staff. These media stereotypes contribute to perpetuating and expanding stigma (see Gabbard and Gabbard, Chapter 11, this volume).

The current role of the psychiatrist in many community mental health facilities adds to the stigmatization. The psychiatrist is often in a position of responsibility with no authority and is the recipient of enmity from other staff members (Clark 1986) (see below under "Current Treatment System").

Adding to the negative image is the accusation that psychiatrists cause or exacerbate mental illness by misdiagnosing patients. That diagnostic label is then inextricable, as are the expectations of "strange" behaviors or dangerousness (Teplin 1985) and society's reaction to the diagnosis. While a misdiagnosis is possible in any field of medicine (e.g., a heart attack that is misdiagnosed as indigestion), the mislabeling that follows the misdiagnosis by a psychiatrist appears to follow the patient and is difficult to deny or eliminate.

Psychiatric nomenclature contributes to this problem. There are no criteria for determining when one is "cured" of schizophrenia. The illness follows one of three patterns: subchronic, in which the symptoms last 6 months to 2 years; chronic, in which symptoms last more than 2 years; or "in remission." There are no criteria for changing the label "in remission" to "no longer mentally disordered." Such a designation would parallel the labeling for cancers. After 5 years of being cancer free, the patient is commonly considered to be "cured," even though the cancer may recur later.

Perceptions of Past Treatments

Past psychiatric treatments often are perceived in a negative light, despite the benefit that many patients have received. Treatments for chronically mentally ill persons have been seen as ineffective, overly harsh, and exacerbating the illness. These impressions have added to the stigma of psychiatrists who work with this population.

Institutional care, the typical treatment for persons who are chronically mentally ill, was designed to provide patients a refuge in a humane, structured environment. However, institutional care has been criticized as being ineffective and, at its worst, as having a negative effect on patients. Patients who remain hospitalized for many years develop a dependency on the numerous services provided by the institution. This "institutionalization syndrome" limits patients' capacity to live independently in the community and has contributed to misgivings about long-term hospitalization of chronically mentally ill persons.

Psychiatrists in this system were assumed to be powerful. They were blamed for promoting dependency and were perceived, by some, as having allowed the deterioration of institutions to occur. In fact, psychiatrists were often one cog in a large bureaucratic system with limited access to funds and little influence on policy (Koz 1979). They were often overwhelmed with large clinical caseloads, which restricted their capacity to influence any one patient's treatment. Psychiatrists were faced with a dilemma. They could remain involved with these institutions and face criticism for their shortcomings, or they could leave the institutions and abandon their patients. Unfortunately, each option reinforced the stigma.

In addition to institutionalization, other past treatments contributed to the stigmatization of psychiatrists who work with persons who are chronically mentally ill. Lobotomies and electroconvulsive therapy (ECT) were seen as being overly harsh and/or destructive. ECT had negative side effects and appeared to be almost barbaric before the use of anesthesia. The actual side effects, along with the image of the process ("zapping a brain"), led to negative perceptions of the entire treatment procedure and to criticism of the psychiatrist who would prescribe such a procedure.

Long-term psychotherapy was considered to be a curative treatment option for chronically mentally ill persons. However, while many patients are helped by psychotherapy, the efficacy of this modality with patients who are chronically mentally ill is currently controversial. Long-term psychotherapy can be harmful to chronically mentally ill persons as a result of the overstimulation and promotion of psychotic regression that occurs (Drake and Sederer 1986). Also, psychotherapy does not "cure" such illnesses as schizophrenia and should not be used instead of medication (Coursey 1989). These acknowledged limitations of psychotherapy contradict earlier treatment assumptions that psychotherapy could be curative with this population. Because therapy did not work, the psychiatrist was seen as ineffective.

Recent approaches to psychotherapy with chronically mentally ill persons are more structured and phenomenological. Three suggested emphases for the therapy are 1) addressing human problems that result from having a psychologically based illness, 2) giving assistance to the patient in managing the illness, and 3) addressing normal psychological problems that arise (Coursey 1989; Ruocchio 1989).

The Current Treatment System

In an effort to remove the "bad" hospital, a new system has been developed that treats the chronically mentally ill patient in the community, thereby eliminating the need for long-term hospitalization. Now, in most parts of the country, brief hospital stays are the norm. This care is perceived by the public to be less restrictive, although concerns remain about recurrent hospitalizations (the "revolving door" syndrome) and the lack of beds for long-term hospitalization. In addition, effective medications are now available. Such procedures as ECT have been improved and now have fewer side effects.

While these current treatments are much improved, the treatment system, with its difficulties and complexities, adds to the stigma toward the psychiatrist of chronically mentally ill patients. Two major concerns appear to impact most on the stigma: the fragmentation of service delivery because of deinstitutionalization and the role the psychiatrist plays in the evolving system.

The fragmentation of service delivery has resulted from the move to deinstitutionalize patients and to serve them in a coordinated care system. However, there are a multiplicity of service-providing systems, including the state, local community mental health centers, hospitals, and independent agencies, that treat such problems as drug and alcohol use, rehabilitation, and housing. The lack of coordination among these services allows people to "slip through the cracks" of the system, as evidenced by the increase in the homeless mentally ill population.

The role of the psychiatrist in the current treatment system is often conflicted. Schindler and associates (1981) found a significant difference between the opinions of psychiatrists and other mental health professionals regarding the competence of psychiatrists to perform evaluation, treatment, and supervision. Psychiatrists felt competent to perform more activities and saw those activities as being part of their role in the treatment system. These perceptions of competence and role were not supported by psychologists and other professionals. The differing perceptions led to rivalry, jealousy, and territoriality, and subsequently to role stress.

Reduced funding (or limited growth in funding) also contributes to the role strain and role conflict. These economic changes have been accompanied by a shift from psychiatric to less expensive treatment staff (Arce and Vergare 1985). In fact, the number of psychiatrists serving in community mental health centers has declined, with a shift from 6.8 full-time psychiatrists per center in 1970 to 3.8 in 1981 (Clark 1986). As other professionals assume more and more of the responsibility for treatment, the psychiatrist is relegated to the role of consultant or pharmacologist. The psychiatrist may have clinical responsibility for several hundred patients. This large a caseload is inconsistent with psychiatric training and traditional roles that teach the psychiatrist to care for the total patient—to be seen as the patient's "doctor." The overwhelming caseload alters the psychiatrist's role to a point at which he or she feels unable to provide adequate care.

Another factor contributing to role strain is the apparent shift of the mission of the community mental health center that occurred during the 1970s—from "medical model/human services" to primarily "human services." The medical mission is to provide psychiatric care for those who cannot pay for private psychiatrists and to provide psychiatric care to those who are chronically mentally ill. The human services mission is to correct social ills that were presumed to be causing mental illness and to treat problems among nonchronically mentally ill community residents (Arce and Vergare 1985). Psychiatrists did not have a clear role in a system assigned to correct social ills, and medical training did not prepare psychiatrists for promoting social change.

Recently, the deemphasis of the state hospital system and the support by the National Alliance for the Mentally Ill (NAMI), other lay organizations, and the organized psychiatric community have led to a remedicalization of services provided to persons who are chronically mentally ill. Role conflicts have been exacerbated as chronically mentally ill patients demand more services, but the time available from psychiatrists continues to be limited.

In order to adjust to the reduced psychiatric resources, the community mental health centers have limited the roles of psychiatrists either to evaluation and dedication prescribing or to consultation with other mental health professionals. The evaluation-remedication role limits participation of the psychiatrist in the treatment life of the patient and can place the physician in a situation in which medication is prescribed for patients not seen by the psychiatrist (Lerro 1974). In the consultation role the psychiatric opinions are rendered without responsibility for patient care. This role is inconsistent with medicolegal and organizational licensing requirements (Arce and Vergare 1985). Thus, the psychiatrist is often left bearing responsibility without authority.

Further, psychiatrists are less often in administrative roles. In fact, the number of community mental health systems run by psychiatrists has declined from 55% in 1970 to 16% in 1985 (Clark 1986). The reduced administrative role of psychiatrists limits participation in decisions regarding the delivery of treatment services. Yet, psychiatrists need access to clinical policy in order to ensure their role in providing medical care (Boyts 1985). However, psychiatrists are often not trained with the range of services that are required for administration (Sherwood et al. 1986; Silver and Marcos 1989).

The changes in the role of the psychiatrist have led to staff enmity, which in turn can lead to a self-fulfilling prophecy. Talented psychiatrists leave the public system when they become discouraged by their limited roles and the attitude of others toward them. Consequently, less capable psychiatrists, newly trained psychiatrists who have yet to establish a private practice, and medical doctors who are not psychiatrists are often left to fill positions in many community mental health centers. Thus, the impression of the incompetent psychiatrist is reinforced by both the restricted role in the community mental health center and the caliber of some psychiatrists who remain in that setting.

Along with the realities of the current treatment system described above are myths that contribute to the stigma of the psychiatrist treating the chronically mentally ill patient. For instance, one myth is that medication leads to cure of the mental illness. Just as people take an antibiotic to clear an infection, many expect that taking medication for a major mental illness will cure that disorder. However, approximately 40% of adequately medicated patients will relapse during the first year of medication (Hogarty 1984).

Even when patients do not relapse, significant impairments persist with optimal psychopharmacological treatment. These impairments include side effects from medication (e.g., tardive dyskinesia). Other symptoms are insensitive to medication. Negative symptoms of schizophrenia tend to be most insensitive to pharmacotherapy. Thus, although most patients do better with pharmacotherapy, the medications currently available do not cure mental illness. The expectation that the medication "should cure" the disorder, and the failure of it to do so, lead to an impression of failure on the part of the psychiatrist prescribing the treatment.

A corollary of this myth is the expectation that patients need only brief and time-limited treatment. When family and community members believe this myth, they are disappointed to discover that treatment continues. The psychiatrist is again blamed for not "curing" the patient in a brief, circumscribed time period. In fact, chronically mentally ill patients require long-term, continuous support.

A second myth focuses on the etiology of the illness. Early theories blamed the "schizophrenic mother" (an idea now repudiated by most modern psychiatrists). Other theories propose that chronic mental illness is a by-product of a pathogenic family system; the deviant behavior is secondary to the pathological interactive system. Family members feel blamed and criticized by proponents of such theories. In order to avoid these feelings of blame, they often hesitate to work with psychiatrists in the treatment of the mentally ill relative. At the professional level, these adversarial feelings have interfered with the formation of a collaborative relationship between psychiatry and family advocates such as those representing the NAMI.

In sum, a number of factors combine to continue the stigma of the psychiatrist treating chronically mentally ill patients in the current treatment system. These include the limited role of the psychiatrist as medicine prescriber or consultant in the community mental health center, staff enmity leading to loss of many talented psychiatrists, myths about treatment outcome, and feelings of blame from family members.

Economics of Care

Current economic constraints imposed on the mental health system discriminate against the severe, complex illnesses that characterize chronically mentally ill persons (Talbott 1988). For instance, arbitrary limits on the length or amount of hospitalization may lead to premature discharges. Critical services, such as psychoeducational programs for the family, vocational services, case management, or special housing arrangements, are not covered under most insurances. As a result of these limitations, patients often receive only a small part of the total services they require. The inadequate funding reflects on psychiatrists who are expected to provide the comprehensive care.

At the state and community levels, underfunding continues. For example, Medicaid fees for outpatient visits in Pennsylvania have not increased from the current level of $25 per hour in 13 years. In addition, the money that went to support the large state hospitals has not followed the patients to the mental health centers or community-based residences (Talbott 1988). Again, without sufficient funds at the federal and state levels, inadequate care is provided; and the psychiatrist often is blamed for the inadequate treatment.

Reducing Stigma

Each of these five factors—patient stigma, the image of the psychiatrist, perceptions of past treatments, the current treatment system, and economics of care—contributes to the stigma of the psychiatrist treating persons who are chronically mentally ill. The interaction of these components multiplies the impact. For example, the image of the psychiatrist treating chronically mentally ill patients is affected by the stereotype of an ineffective, undervalued professional. This stereotype is reinforced through a treatment system that minimizes the role of the psychiatrist and through biases about older treatments and a limited understanding of current treatment capabilities (e.g., understanding that medication and hospitalization are not cures for chronic mental illness) among the general public.

Having described the interactive components of stigmatization, the next step is to determine activities that will impact on that model to decrease the stigma. Because the components are interactive, stigma can be decreased by modifying any component in the model. However, some components are more easily changed than others, and some of these changes will have greater impact than others. In general, broad attempts to educate the public against the stereotypical view of mentally ill individuals (patient stigma) or about past psychiatric treatment (perceptions of past treatment) are likely to be slow processes at best. The stigma attributed to mentally ill persons is particularly difficult to dislodge because the media continuously reconfirm the stereotypes.

Perceptions of past treatments are not likely to change. To some degree, the concerns raised about these treatment strategies are appropriate. The large institutions were fraught with problems, and such treatments as lobotomies did have negative side effects.

Much progress has been made in the treatment of persons who are chronically mentally ill. Model community treatment programs are maximizing patients' independence through the use of flexible coordination of an array of outpatient community resources. Families are being taught to cope and adapt to the problems engendered by living with a chronically mentally ill relative. New medications are being used to treat formerly resistant patients. However, the current treatment system does have some limitations that must be recognized and presented to the family. These include the facts that treatment is long-term and has accompanying side effects, and there is likely to be relapse despite compliance to recommended medical regimens.

We recommend specific actions that are likely to have a greater impact on changing the image of the psychiatrist who treats chronically mentally ill patients. First, as a professional group, psychiatrists must lobby to effect changes in the economics of care. Increased funding is needed for programming in community mental health centers and for increases in the number of psychiatrists at these centers. Salary increases are also necessary to attract quality staff at every level of service delivery. Raising salaries is a direct means of destigmatizing this professional group, since salary is related to status. Higher salaries and better-funded programs will attract and maintain higher caliber psychiatrists in the public sector. In this way the self-fulfilling prophecies described earlier will be reversed.

Funds are also needed to increase the research on current treatment for the chronically mentally ill patient population in order to develop more effective treatment protocols. Along with the need for research funding is the necessity to integrate programs in universities and medical schools. In Maryland, for example, a system-to-system relationship has been established between the state mental hospitals and the University of Maryland School of Medicine. Psychiatrists treating chronically mentally ill persons have appointments in the university, residents train in both facilities, and psychiatrists participate in administrative meetings (Talbott 1988). This hospital-university interaction facilitates research and increases interprofessional contacts. The association also helps to decrease the stigma of the psychiatrist treating patients who are chronically mentally ill.

In addition, changes in the current treatment system are needed. Roles need to be modified in order to reduce role strain experienced by psychiatrists who work with chronically mentally ill persons. Psychiatrists have traditionally served two general roles: direct care to the chronically mentally ill patients in state hospital or community mental health center settings, and administration. Each of these roles will be considered separately along with recommendations for changes that might reduce the stigma associated with psychiatrists in these roles.

The direct care role in the community mental health center setting is important because the center is the most likely site for the provision of clinical services to chronically mentally ill patients in the near future. In addition, the current emphasis on the biologic underpinnings of chronic mental illness has reinforced the need for psychiatric involvement in treatment. Simultaneously, there has been recognition that patients require a broad range of services including rehabilitation, involvement of family, education, and housing. The role of the psychiatrist has become unclear because it is difficult to differentiate medical treatment from social services. For instance, when family and staff plan for the care of a suicidal patient it is unclear whether such planning is primarily a social (social worker) or medical (psychiatrist) responsibility. This lack of clarity is unavoidable, and leadership is required that can encompass many disciplines.

Because of their breadth of training and experiences with persons who are chronically mentally ill and with the systems they utilize, psychiatrists are in a unique position to resolve the ambiguity by taking a leadership role within the treatment system. Psychiatric training provides an understanding of the normal and pathological functioning of biological systems in man. In addition, this training provides the skills for analysis of psychological and social systems, the ability to traverse different frames of reference, and the capacity to integrate humanistic and scientific approaches to health care (Eisen 1986). The suggestion that psychiatrists assume positions of leadership in the treatment of chronically mentally ill patients is controversial because of the overlap between disciplines involved. However, such leadership is necessary in order to prevent interminable interprofessional conflict and to maintain the prominence of the medical aspects of treatment.

In order for psychiatrists to assume that leadership responsibility, they need to be trained in skills necessary for competent leadership. Appropriate training provides knowledge, clinical skills, and experience in treating this population. Curriculum guidelines for the training of residents to work within the community mental health system have recently been published (Faulkner et al. 1989).

The second role of the psychiatrist in treating chronically mentally ill patients is that of administrator. Some authors have suggested that the decreasing psychiatric involvement in community mental health center administration should continue. Training physicians to fulfill administrative tasks is expensive and complex (Sherwood et al. 1986). However, I believe that the administrative role is essential for the psychiatrist in the community mental health center system. This involvement allows for input into the development, implementation, and maintenance of clinical policy. Psychiatric involvement in policy reduces conflicts that impede patient care (Boyts 1985), and integrates medical and psychosocial aspects of care. Such integration is necessary as the complexity of care for patients who are chronically mentally ill increases. In addition, care is being more closely regulated by government and influenced by business interests. Psychiatric training offers the necessary knowledge to determine a clinical policy that integrates these multiple factors and arrives at scientific and humanistic patient care.

Some of the responsibilities of the psychiatrist as an administrator include medical screening, supervision of other physicians, assuring quality of psychiatric services, and developing educational programs. An important aspect of the administrative role is working with the executive officer to develop and review programs and budgets. Also, the administrative psychiatrist might work as the liaison with other hospitals and medical personnel.

Administrative responsibilities should also be a part of residency training. Residents need to recognize the value of the administrative role and to understand the leadership contribution of psychiatry to the interdisciplinary clinical treatment team. Also, psychiatric residents should understand the impact of clinical decisions and policy on treatment.

The role of the psychiatrist cannot be generated de novo within every community mental health center. Coordination and influence of national organizations is necessary to develop an appropriate role for professionals. Without national guidelines, roles will remain variable and conflictual. The combination of training and institutional support can help to define a role for the psychiatrist that is less stigmatized.

Stigma can also be reduced if psychiatrists network with family advocates, patient advocates, other mental health professionals and government officials involved in mental health care. In Philadelphia, under the auspices of Paul Jay Fink, M.D., we have set up such a network. Representatives from the Philadelphia Psychiatric Society, Pennsylvania and local Alliance for the Mentally Ill, and the Mental Health Association (including patient advocates and government officials) have met one evening per month for the past 2 years. These meetings have promoted communication among these groups. Misconceptions, such as the belief that psychiatry blames families for causing schizophrenia, can be corrected. Advocates gain a more realistic appraisal of psychiatrists' limitations. And psychiatrists hear, first-hand, advocates' concerns. Legal initiatives, such as pending legislation, are discussed in order to coordinate the efforts of each organization. Some differences can be resolved. However, when genuine differences of opinion or interest occur, they are discussed in an atmosphere of mutual respect. In addition to reducing stigma by reducing distortions and promoting communication, these meetings have spurred the interest of professional psychiatric organizations to address the needs of persons who are chronically mentally ill.

In sum, by lobbying for funds for treatment and for research, affiliating psychiatrists who treat chronically mentally ill patients with universities, increasing residency training to address treatment of chronic mental illness and to include administrative skills, redefining the role of the psychiatrists in the treatment system for patients who are chronically mentally ill, and working with patient and family advocates, we can impact on the stigma of the psychiatrist treating this special population.

References

Andreasen N: Scale for the Assessment of Negative Symptoms. Iowa City, IA, The University of Iowa (Nancy C Andreasen), 1984

Arce AA, Vergare MJ: Psychiatrists and interprofessional role in community mental health centers, in Community Mental Health Centers and Psychiatrists. Washington, DC, American Psychiatric Association; Rockville, MD, National Council of Community Mental Health Centers, 1985, pp 51–68

Boyts H: Overview—recruiting and retaining psychiatrists to work in community mental health centers: overcoming the obstacles, in Community Mental Health Centers and Psychiatrists. Washington, DC, American Psychiatric Association; MD, National Council of Community Mental Health Centers, 1985, pp 7–21

Clark GH Jr: Community Psychiatry: Problems and Possibilities. Spring House, PA, McNeil Pharmaceutical, 1986

Coursey RD: Psychotherapy with persons suffering from schizophrenia: the need for a new agenda. Schizophr Bull 15:349–353, 1989

Drake RE, Sederer LI: The adverse effects of intensive treatment of chronic schizophrenia. Compr Psychiatry 27:313–326, 1986

Eisen P: Potential for psychiatric leadership in health care. Aust N Z J Psychiatry 20:107–111, 1986

Faulkner LR, Cutler DL, Krohn DD, et al: A basic residency curriculum concerning the chronically mentally ill. Am J Psychiatry 146:1323–1327, 1989

Hogarty GE: Depot neuroleptics: the relevance of psychosocial factors—a United States perspective. J Clin Psychiatry 45(5):36–41, 1984

Jones EE, Farina A, Hastorf AH, et al: Social Stigma: The Psychology of Marked Relationships. New York, WH Freeman, 1984

Koz G: Catch 22: the psychiatrist in the state hospital. Psychiatric Annals 9:47–54, 1979

Lerro FA: Potential problems facing psychiatrists in mental health centers. Hosp Community Psychiatry 25:808, 1974

Ruocchio PJ: How psychotherapy can help the schizophrenic patient. Hosp Community Psychiatry 40:188–190, 1989

Schindler RE, Berren MR, Beigel A: A study of the causes of conflict between psychiatrists and psychologists. Hosp Community Psychiatry 32:263–266, 1981

Sherwood E, Greenblatt M, Pasnau RO: Psychiatric residency, role models, and leadership. Am J Psychiatry 143:764, 1986

Silver MA, Marcos LR: The making of the psychiatrist-executive. Am J Psychiatry 146:29–34, 1989

Talbott JA: The Perspective of John Talbott. San Francisco, CA, Jossey-Bass, 1988

Teplin LA: The criminality of the mentally ill: a dangerous misconception. Am J Psychiatry 142:593–599, 1985

Chapter 19

Overcoming Stigma:
The Mad Hatters

One of the most potent methods of combating stigma of the past decade has been the development of theatrical groups, often comprised of recovered or recovering mentally ill persons and/or theatrical professionals, who deal with the subject of stigma in a highly emotionally charged way.

The Mad Hatters is a disability organization of theater and human services professionals. Through dramatic performances, the group sets the stage for integration of people with disabilities. Professionals and community members with disabilities are actively involved on the staff and board of The Mad Hatters. During the 1989 annual meeting of the American Psychiatric Association in San Francisco, their performance was very well received. The following describes their growth, mission, and technique.

Kalamazoo, Michigan is a mid-sized city with a thriving downtown business community. One of Kalamazoo's claims to fame is the city's possession of the United States' first open-air mall. This mall, located in the heart of Kalamazoo's business district, is a wonderful community resource. People congregate in the Kalamazoo mall during lunch hour on weekdays, teenagers spend time on the mall, Kalamazoo residents shop and visit there, mothers take their children out in strollers for promenades down the mall. This is an area that is generally seen to be a safe and friendly environment for socializing, errand running, taking care of business, relaxing, dining, and taking in the fresh air on one's lunch hour. However, in 1979, Kalamazoo's business district had serious concerns about the future vitality of the mall, due to the arrival of numerous former residents of the Kalamazoo Regional Psychiatric Hospital (KRPH).

In 1979 when many residents of KRPH were deinstitutionalized, the Kalamazoo County Board of Mental Health conducted a survey to explore how Kalamazoo residents felt about sharing their community with these people who had been released from the hospital. Results from this survey revealed that people were apprehensive, concerned, awkward, and sometimes fearful toward these former state hospital residents.

217

The Mad Hatters was created to address these concerns in a creative way that would gently and gradually ask people to examine their feelings and attitudes and, if possible, restructure them in more positive directions. The vehicle chosen to effect this change was drama, because of its power to reach people on an emotional level. Diverse professionals from the fields of education, theater, and human services pooled their expertise to create an educational theater with a mission: to foster improved understanding, acceptance, and social inclusion of people with special needs. Not a simple task, for society's citizens with special needs have long been outcasts in one way or another. It took the movement to bring these "differently abled" persons out of the institutions, where they had been virtually invisible, and into their communities to reveal a formidable obstacle in this process of transition.

Stigma is the most debilitating of all the problems encountered by people with special needs or disabilities in striving to live lives of involvement and meaning within their communities. The Mad Hatters Educational Theatre for the Understanding of People With Special Needs or Disabilities has created a unique model for dispelling the myths and stereotypes that so limit persons who are physically, emotionally, or mentally challenged. This model combines sensitive dramas, artistic portrayals, and direct audience interaction with the actor(s) in character, led by a trained program facilitator. Audience members are given the opportunity to spend time talking with people with many different disabilities. By simply talking with the characters, discomfort is alleviated and understanding is deepened.

The Mad Hatters has come a long way. Dedication, hard work, and the generosity of those who support that work have paid off, allowing The Mad Hatters to grow from a totally volunteer organization in 1979 into a fully staffed professional theater company offering over 100 performances nationwide in 1989. Growth in recent years has been phenomenal, from 43 performances in 1985 to 107 performances in 1989. In 1989 over 15,000 people across the country participated in performances by The Mad Hatters in audiences that ranged from 50 to 1,000 people in size. This growth rate has been accompanied by heightened visibility and national recognition. Recent performances at national conferences have included those of the Council for Exceptional Children, the President's Committee for Employment of Persons With Disabilities, and the American Psychiatric Association. In 1990 The Mad Hatters offered approximately 120 performances to national and international audiences totaling an estimated 19,000 people. In December 1989, The Mad Hatters completed Phase I of the training of a pilot troupe for model replication in Bermuda.

The future holds increasing levels of state, national, and international touring, the possibility of training more troupes in the United States and in other countries, and exploration of employing drama to combat the stigma surrounding persons with disabilities in a video or film medium.

Video as an Agent of Attitude Change?

In 1989, The Mad Hatters produced and field tested a video, *The Wish List*, to compare its power to effect with other presentational methods positive attitudinal change toward people who have disabilities. Results of this field testing, conducted in fourth- and fifth-grade classrooms in the Kalamazoo Public Schools, show that the most effective method of promoting positive attitude change toward persons with disabilities is brought about by direct interaction with people who are disabled, as the literature supports. The other methods that were involved in this comparison study included a lecture on disabilities, a live dramatic presentation in which actors who were not disabled portrayed disabled characters and directly interacted with the students, a video presentation in which the students viewed *The Wish List*, and a control group that received no intervention. No conclusive statistical evidence was found to support the use of the lecture or video models as agents of change at the 1-month post-test; there was statistically significant positive change for those students who participated in the live dramatic and the live panel presentations. No statistical evidence was found at the 1-month post-test to indicate that the live theater model was a more effective agent of change than the video and the lecture models, which showed no significant change at the 1-month post-test.

The Mad Hatters is hopeful of finding more conclusive evidence to support the medium of video as an agent of positive attitude change toward persons with disabilities because of the greater audience that can be reached through this venue.

How Stigma Limits Persons With Disabilities

There are tangible obstacles to full social inclusion of the "differently abled." Physical barriers can impede the accessibility of buildings and modes of transportation. Physically, mentally, or emotionally challenged people do indeed find some aspects of their lives much more challenging than do the rest of us who are "temporarily able." What people with disabilities find to be the greatest challenge in striving to live integrated and involved lives in their communities is not, however, the limitations placed upon them by their physical environment or their physical or mental impairments. The greatest challenge lies in the necessity to confront, day after day, the fear, the discomfort, and the negative attitudes of the vast majority of the general public when interacting with people who have disabilities.

It is not long before carrying the weight of such a social stigma begins to have its effect. Despite great effort and ability, a person with a disability has great difficulty to find an accepting employer who will offer him or her a job. It is hard to continue to try in the face of the palpable discomfort or fear or insensitivity of others. Negative public attitude has resulted in America's largest minority—an estimated 36 million people who have disabilities—feeling a loss in self-worth, frightened of rejection, and living in isolation.

These negative attitudes on the part of the general public are ill-founded. People with disabilities need not bear the burden of social stigma. The public must be better informed about the issues faced by people with special needs. Only by dispelling the myths and stereotypes that have so limited people with disabilities in the past can people with disabilities be free to pursue meaningful lives. Through broader exposure to the people behind the disabilities, community acceptance, understanding, and integration can become a reality. Discrimination is a fact of life for people with disabilities. This needs to change.

Counteracting Stigma With Educational Theater: The Mad Hatters

For 10 years, The Mad Hatters has been employing theater to convey its message of social integration for people with special needs or disabilities. The power of drama to elicit profound audience response is remarkable. Through drama, The Mad Hatters is able to lead audience members to examine their attitudes toward people with disabilities and heighten their awareness of how these attitudes impact upon the lives of people with special needs.

Each performance consists of a number of short vignettes designed to give audience members poignant glances of the people behind the disabling conditions. Audience members are encouraged to ask characters questions and are brought to realize that many of their own feelings, hopes, frustrations, dreams, and fears are shared by these people whom they had perceived as being so very different from themselves. This realization is achieved through the intervention of a skilled audience facilitator who works with the actor in character to guide audience participants toward greater understanding and acceptance of people who are "differently abled."

Each audience member is encouraged to don a hat as the performance begins. The hats are offered as the audience's invitation to participate—to enter the lives of the disabled characters they meet and transcend the barriers between actor and audience—between people who are strangers to one another—and take a moment to care and consider the needs of people with disabilities. "Differently abled" persons' needs are not so special. These persons need acceptance, affection, support, understanding, employment, and approbation for their particular qualities and efforts. The Mad Hatters is able to give audience members the opportunity to witness the similarities behind the difference for the disabled and the "temporarily able." Through a model that is powerful, a vital message is conveyed with a lasting positive impact on the quality of life for people who have disabilities.

Objectives

Stated simply, The Mad Hatters' mission is to foster improved understanding, acceptance, and societal inclusion of people who are disabled. Theater enables The Mad Hatters to involve audience participants at an emotional level. In directly involving audience participants with actors who are portraying disabled characters, The Mad Hatters is working to promote positive attitude change toward persons with disabilities. Attitude change is a very difficult thing to measure—and to infer ensuing behavioral change is assuming causality, which is something this organization is not prepared to do. What The Mad Hatters believes is that it sets the stage for change.

Testimony from past audience participants indicates that paving the path for change is valuable in dispelling the stigma that so limits people who are disabled. Examples of such testimony include the special education teacher who wrote to The Mad Hatters some time after a Mad Hatters performance for regular and special educators in her school district to report that as the result of this performance, the school district revised the way it conducted its individual Educational Planning Committees (EPCs) for special education students. As another example, a woman who had attended a Mad Hatters performance addressing employment of persons with disabilities wrote to say that because of the performance she had promoted one disabled employee and hired another.

The list of testimonies is a long one. While The Mad Hatters does not take the credit for such changes, it is possible that performances by The Mad Hatters increase the likelihood that people will positively change their attitudes toward persons with disabilities. Setting the stage for the lessening of the stigma that surrounds persons with disabilities in American society is how The Mad Hatters works to foster improved acceptance, understanding, and social inclusion of the "differently abled."

Evaluation of Objectives and Programming

The method of evaluating the objectives listed above as well as the overall quality of The Mad Hatters programming consists of four steps:

1. Distribution of performance evaluation forms to each audience member at each performance
2. Mailing follow-up evaluation forms to audience members who have provided their names and addresses
3. Tabulation and analysis of both the immediate and the follow-up evaluations
4. Documentation of responses

The immediate performance evaluation is a checklist of items that measures the artistic quality and educational value of the performance, as well as audience members' personal feelings and perceptions. Written comments are also invited, and overall ratings range from poor to excellent.

Follow-up evaluations are mailed approximately 4 months after each performance. The purpose of these evaluations is to solicit from past audience members examples of specific attitude and/or behavior changes that have resulted from participating in The Mad Hatters performance.

Immediate evaluations are tabulated and summarized by computer, creating percentages and frequency of response to each item on the checklist. Each follow-up evaluation is read and analyzed by the director of The Mad Hatters and entered into a monthly report summarizing specific attitude and behavior changes. All evaluation summaries are kept on file and are available for reporting purposes.

The Mad Hatters is seeking more effective and objective methods of finding evidence to document that participation in a Mad Hatters performance can begin to lessen the stigma that unfortunately so often accompanies a disability. Many hours of discussion with evaluation professionals have taken place, and several changes are being considered in exploring ways to demonstrate more successfully the impact of a Mad Hatters performance. As of yet, no solid decisions have been made. What The Mad Hatters can definitively claim is that it is an organization that carries a positive message to the public about inclusion of persons with disabilities. What cannot be stated yet is that this positive message effects positive attitude change. A review of the literature, however, reveals that there is reason to believe that this could be so. It is The Mad Hatters' hope that future research and evaluation will continue to enforce and more strongly support the hypothesis of this theater; that The Mad Hatters dramatic model can set the stage for positive attitudinal change toward persons with disabilities, and so augment the potential for a higher quality of life for this population that presently bears the burden of social stigma.

The Impact of Drama on Attitudes and Behaviors Toward People With Special Needs or Disabilities: Review of the Literature

Research supports the use of role playing or disability simulation as one way of producing a positive shift in public attitudes toward people with disabilities. Closer examination of this research yields further support for the use of drama and the dramatic process, such as the unique interactive model used by The Mad Hatters, as a powerful agent for effecting directed attitudinal change.

Current Attitudes and Attitude Change

Negative public attitude has historically been one of the greatest obstacles preventing individuals with special needs or disabilities from leading more productive, meaningful, and involved lives in modern society. Although recent legislation has mandated increased integration and equal opportunity for this country's disabled population, the outcome of such action is entirely dependent upon the American public and its willingness, ability, and opportunity to see beyond labels and visible differences to the inner human characteristics that make us all more like one another than different.

The consequences of the general public's current negative attitudes toward persons with disabilities continue to greatly limit and discriminate against an estimated 36 million Americans who are disabled. McKalip (1979, p. 293) states, "Listed among virtually every psychologist's list of human needs is the need to be accepted, the need to belong." Rather than being accepted and feeling as though they belong, however, persons who are disabled far too often must struggle with their own fear of rejection and feelings of shame or inferiority (Link et al. 1987), low self-esteem (Gresham et al. 1988), and social isolation (Riester and Bessette 1986).

Attitudes toward people with disabilities have been the focus of much research during the last quarter century. Studies attempting to identify effective methods of modifying these attitudes have been conducted and have yielded a set of varied results that, in one author's words, "leaves the professional or advocate who desires to produce attitude change somewhat bewildered" (Donaldson 1980, p 505). In a comprehensive analysis of these studies in which he identifies those factors that produce positive attitude change and which techniques can be easily employed and replicated, Donaldson (1980, pp. 505–508) reaches the following conclusions:

1. Structured experiences with or presentations by disabled persons consistently resulted in positive attitude change ...
2. Nonstereotypic attitudes are more likely to emerge when disabled and non-disabled persons are of at least equal status ...
3. Formation of positive attitudes and/or the reduction of discomfort and avoidance behavior may ... be closely associated with careful exposure to disabled persons who do not themselves act in a stereotypic manner
4. No direct cause or relationship probably exists between the provision of limited information about disabilities and attitude change ...
5. Results which yielded negative shifts in attitudes suggest caution in the use of unstructured group discussion ...
6. Role-playing and the vicarious experience of observing that role-playing were effective methods of modifying at least some dimensions of attitudes toward disability ...

Similarly, McKalip (1979, p. 294) identifies three steps that are necessary in "training individuals to accept differences among people":

1. Develop or enhance people's ability to empathize . . .
2. Provide the opportunity for people to examine their attitudes, feelings, and actions, focusing on empathizing.
3. Provide exposure to handicapped individuals in a positive environment where non-handicapped people can receive unbiased information.

Clark (1930) supports McKalip's conviction about the importance of empathy in accepting differences. He states that "one of the most effective means of removing prejudice is found in the process of identification, of putting oneself in the place of the other fellow" (p. 56). Setting up a positive environment for the exploration of differences by creating a simulation exercise can encourage empathy. Interviewing a nonhandicapped person sitting in a wheelchair is one way to role-play. After explaining the person's disability, then ask questions such as, "What do you do for fun?" Observers of the role playing are affected similarly to those actually involved.

Drama and Its Impact

At various times throughout history, drama has been employed for reasons other than purely aesthetic ones. The early Greeks used theater "to express the dilemmas of the human condition" (Davis 1987, p. 301) . In the 1940s, Joseph Moreno brought theater back to that original form with the development of psychodrama, a form of psychotherapy employing dramatic techniques. Most recently, drama has come to play a unique role in human psychology and sociology through the emergence of drama therapy as a professionally recognized treatment approach. Examples of successful projects, both in practice as well as in research, support the use of drama in creating an environment for healthy change. Alban Metcalfe (1984) reports that in a controlled study measuring the use of drama in teaching science, greater meaningful learning occurred when drama was used. In addition, many theater professionals across the nation are currently coupling their art with various areas of social concern, as documented by Burnham (1988). Some of these organizations and the issues they address include the Theatre Workers Project in Los Angeles (unemployment); the Boulder Arts Workshop (biculturalism); Artists Confronting AIDS; and Hospital Audiences in New York (elderly and mental illness). As Burnham states, "Perhaps what these artists are proving about the function of art is that it is a vehicle for spiritual and social transformation" (p. 39).

What is it about drama that makes it such a positive agent with which to stimulate change? Polsky (1976; cited in Davis 1987, p. 299) asserts that "because the essence of drama is human conflict, enacting dramatic situations enables the participants to deal with the process of confrontation and thus in a controlled setting have the freedom to express feelings which might otherwise go untapped." Regarding the development of psychodrama, Davis (1987) reports that "[Joseph] Moreno perceived one important therapeutic spin-off of psychodrama to be the release of spontaneity, which enabled participants to deal creatively with new life situations, rather than reacting in stereotyped, non-productive patterns" (p. 300). McLeod (1984) explains this relatively recent movement in modern psychology, citing Fromm's (1956) notion of "collective art," illustrated by such communal events as religious rituals, dance, passion plays, and Greek drama. "Such groups," states McLeod, "are certainly places where people come together, outside the routine of everyday life, to participate in emotionally involving interactions in which existential value orientations are illustrated by means of dramatic interplay" (p. 321). In his discussion of similarities between the stages of group processing and those found in typical plot development, McLeod writes,

> both ... move into a stage of exploration of feelings and relationships, often involving a degree of conflict. Both end with a period during which issues are cleared up, business is completed, changes in behavior or attitudes are witnessed or reported, and the outside world is re-engaged. (p. 323)

Of particular interest here is the effect of drama not only on participants (i.e., actors) but also on the audience. Scheff (1979) maintains that the role of the actor is to create in the audience a balanced emotional state or "an aesthetic distance." McLeod (1984, p. 326) summarizes Scheff's suggestion that "when individuals are both participating in and observing their own emotions, it becomes possible for them to go through a process of catharsis by which previously repressed emotional experiences ... can be expressed and lived through." Indeed research on attitude change indicates that observers as well as participants are positively affected by their involvement in simulation or role-playing exercises (McKalip 1979; Wilson and Alcorn 1969).

This process of audience self-examination is supported by Drummond (1984) and Furman (1988) in their respective discussions of audience participation and "distancing" theories as applied to the theater. Indeed, as Furman notes, "the theater audience itself is an appropriate group for the therapeutic experience" (p. 245).

The Use of Drama to Change Attitudes

Returning to the previously mentioned factors that effectively promote positive attitude change toward people with disabilities, it is clear that the use of drama incorporates these factors, providing an effective and easily replicated technique. The development of empathy through examination of one's own attitudes or behaviors (McKalip 1979), structured contact with disabled persons (Evans 1976; Langor et al. 1976; Lazar et al. 1971; Sedlick and Penta 1975), and simulation exercises (McKalip 1979; Wilson and Alcorn 1969) have all been identified as successful methods of facilitating attitude change. Participation as an audience member in a dramatic model provides the opportunity for structured contact through simulation, which creates increased empathy and can result in a positive shift in attitudes.

Interaction between actors simulating or portraying disabled characters and audience members provides exposure or contact in a structured setting, where disabled and nondisabled persons are of equal status and where disabled persons do not necessarily act in a stereotypical manner. The audience, if allowed to reach its emotional balance and thereby create an "aesthetic distance," responds to that interaction by examining and expressing feelings "which might otherwise go untapped" (Polsky 1976; cited in Davis 1987, p. 299). As a result, "changes in attitudes are witnessed or reported, and the outside world is re-engaged" (McLeod 1984, p. 323).

Conclusion

The Mad Hatters, Theatre for the Understanding of People With Special Needs or Disabilities, has been refining the technique of employing educational theater to promote positive attitude and behavior change toward persons with disabilities for a decade. Founded in 1980, The Mad Hatters continues to receive testimony that strongly supports the use of this theater's model in effecting positively directed attitude change on the part of the audience participants toward persons with disabilities.

References

Alban Metcalfe RJ, et al: Teaching science through drama: an empirical investigation. Research in Science and Technological Education 2(1):77–81, 1984

Anthony WA: The effects of contact on an individual's attitude toward disabled persons. Rehabilitation Counseling Bulletin 12:168–170, 1969

Burnham LR: Tracking a new wave of socially committed art. American Theatre, August 1988, pp 38–40

Clark EL: The Art of Straight Thinking. New York, D Appleton, 1930

Davis BW: Some roots of relatives of creative drama as an enrichment activity for older adults. Educational Gerontology 13:297–306, 1987

Donaldson J: Changing attitudes toward handicapped persons: a review and analysis of research. Exceptional Children 46:504–514, 1980

Drummond J: The theatregoer as imager. Journal of Mental Imagery 8:99–104, 1984

Evans JH: Changing attitudes toward disabled persons: an experimental study. Rehabilitation Counseling Bulletin 19:572–579, 1976

Fromm E: The Sane Society. London, Routledge & Kegan Paul, 1956

Furman L: Theatre as therapy: the distancing effect applied to audience. Arts in Psychotherapy 15:245–249, 1988

Gresham FM, Evans SN: Self-efficacy differences among mildly handicapped, gifted, and nonhandicapped students. Journal of Special Education 22:231–240, 1988

Kent D, Cater E: The origin and development of psychodrama and its relationship to radical theatre. Group Psychotherapy and Psychodrama 27:71–82, 1974–1975

Langor EJ, Fiske S, Taylor SE, et al: Stigma, sharing and discomfort: a novel-stimulus hypothesis. Journal of Experimental Social Psychology 12:451–463, 1976

Lazar AL, Gensley JT, Orpet RE: Changing attitudes of young mentally gifted children toward handicapped persons. Exceptional Children 37:600–602, 1971

Link BG, Cullen FT, Frank J, et al: The social rejection of former mental patients: understanding why labels matter. American Journal of Sociology 92:1461–1500, 1987

Marsh V, Friedman R: Changing public attitudes toward blindness. Exceptional Children 38:426–428, 1972

McKalip KJ: Developing acceptance toward the handicapped. School Counselor 26:293–298, 1979

McLeod J: Group process as drama. Small Group Behavior 15:319–332, 1984

Polsky M: The Brookdale Drama Project. New York, Hunter College, Department of Theatre and Cinema, Brookdale Center on Aging, 1976

Rapier J, Adelson R, Carey R, et al: Changes in children's attitudes toward the physically handicapped. Exceptional Children 39:212–219, 1972

Riester AE, Bessette KM: Preparing the peer group for mainstreaming exceptional children. Pointer 31(1):12–20, 1986

Scheff TJ: Catharsis in Healing, Ritual, and Drama. Santa Barbara, CA, University of California Press, 1979

Sedlick M, Penta JB: Changing nurse attitudes toward quadriplegics through use of television. Rehabilitation Literature 36:274–278, 288, 1975

Seltzer MM: Differential impact of various experiences on breaking down age stereotypes. Educational Gerontology 2:183–189, 1977

Siperstein GN, Bak JJ, Gottlieb J: Effects of group discussion on children's attitudes toward handicapped peers. Journal of Educational Research 70:131–134, 1977

Wilson EE, Alcorn D: Disability simulation and development of attitudes toward the exceptional. Journal of Special Education 3:303–307, 1969

Index

(Bold type denotes table)